CW00675031

THE YOGA SŪTRAS OF PATAÑJALI

THE YOGA SŪTRAS OF PATAÑJALI

THE OXFORD CENTRE FOR HINDU STUDIES GUIDE

NICHOLAS SUTTON

A RECOGNISED INDEPENDENT CENTRE OF THE UNIVERSITY OF OXFORD

The Oxford Centre for Hindu Studies
The Yoga Sūtras of Patañjali

Copyright © 2017 by Oxford Centre for Hindu Studies

Published by the Oxford Centre for Hindu Studies
13-15 Magdalen St, Oxford OX1 3AE, UK

www.ochsonline.org
Regd Charity No. 1074458

ISBN 978-1-5272-1037-0

CONTENTS

INTRODUCTION

✻

THIS short book provides a detailed consideration of what is perhaps the best known, but least well understood, of all the texts of Indian philosophy, the *Yoga Sūtras* of Patañjali. This is not a particularly easy text to study, nor one where the meaning can be easily understood. The *Yoga Sūtras* exists within the context of early Indian philosophy, which is in itself a highly complex and at times obscure area of study, and the comprehension of its principal tenets becomes even more problematic without some knowledge of that wider context.

I would certainly not try to discourage anyone from taking up such a study, however, and I do believe that an understanding of Patañjali's work at any level is a prerequisite for acquiring a proper insight into the philosophy of Yoga. I do feel, however, that too much is written and said about the *Yoga Sūtras* that is not based on a thorough reading of the text, and as a result tends to be misleading. Hence in writing a study guide to the *Yoga Sūtras*, one inevitably encounters a tension between on the one hand making the ideas accessible to as many readers as possible, and, on the other, doing full justice to the complexity of the ideas encountered. Whether or not I have the balance right is for others to judge, but I do hope the reader will appreciate the difficulties involved in introducing this text as an area of study.

Taking a more positive note, I would certainly say that anyone who goes through this study guide will emerge both enriched and enlightened, and with a much deeper understanding of the Yoga tradition. That is not to say that I expect everyone to immediately understand every part of the *Sūtras*, as that would be highly unlikely, merely that even a partial or imperfect comprehension will be of enormous benefit in gaining an understanding of the philosophy of Yoga.

DATE AND AUTHORSHIP OF THE YOGA SŪTRAS

Although he does not name himself in the text, the identity of a certain Patañjali as the author of the *Yoga Sūtras* is well attested. Despite legends about his birth and identity, we can say little for certain about who he was or indeed about when he lived. According to popular accounts, Patañjali is supposed to be a manifestation of the divine serpent Ananta who acts as the bed of Viṣṇu. Ananta appeared on earth to disseminate knowledge of Yoga and because he fell (*pata*) into the hands of his mother whilst they were formed into the position of prayer (*añjali*), he was given the name of Patañjali.

In more historical terms, the debate over the dating of the text rests substantially on whether the author of the *Yoga Sūtras* is to be identified as the grammarian named Patañjali, who probably lived in the 2nd century BC. Indian traditions seem to take this identity for granted but most modern scholars are more sceptical, and suggest that our Patañjali probably lived some time in the 2nd or 3rd centuries AD. It is virtually impossible to be certain on this matter, but it does appear that the *Yoga Sūtras* has an awareness of the *Bhagavad-gītā*, and on this basis alone the later date is perhaps more likely. I would also tentatively suggest that the *Yoga* Sūtras should be regarded as being later than the passages from the *Mahābhārata* which focus on Yoga practice and the philosophy of Yoga.

THE STATUS OF THE YOGA SŪTRAS

Hindu religious thought recognises six *darśanas,* or philosophical systems, as orthodox. These six, Ved*ā*nta, Mīm*ā*ṁsa,

Vaiśeṣika, Nyāya, Sāṁkhya and Yoga, are declared to be orthodox, or *āstika*, because they accept the Vedic revelation as authoritative. Those systems that do not accept the authority of the Veda are said to be *na āstika*, or *nāstika*, and are frequently condemned in Hindu texts; these would include Buddhists, Jains, and Ājīvikas, as well as the more overtly atheist philosophies such as the Cārvākas and Lokāyatas. Each of the *āstika* systems has a defining text, which purports to establish its fundamental principles. Most of these are written in the *sūtra* style of pithy aphorisms, which generally require a commentary or verbal explanation for the full meaning to become clear; the *Sāṁkhya Kārikā* is the one exception to this rule.

With regard to the Yoga *darśana*, Patañjali's *Yoga Sūtras* holds the position of being the seminal work that defines the system, and for this reason alone it appears to have always been held in high regard; even today, when Yoga has progressed considerably from the teachings of Patañjali, it is still usually referred to as the principal work on Yoga with authoritative status. Over the centuries a number of important commentaries have been written, which seek to explain and extrapolate the full meaning of the *sūtras*. The earliest of these commentaries is that of Vyasa, who is sometimes identified with the legendary author of the *Mahābhārata* and compiler of the Veda, although this seems highly unlikely, and most scholars suggest a date some time between the 5th and 8th centuries AD. Other important writers on the *Yoga Sūtras* include the great Vedāntist, Vācaspati Miśra (10th century), Bhoja the philosopher king of Malwa in central India (11th century), and Vijñānabhikṣu (16th century), who challenged Śaṅkarācārya's philosophy of Advaita Vedānta.

It would require a great deal of study to look in detail at the commentarial tradition, but the fact that these different works exist shows again the high regard in which the *Yoga Sūtras* was held. In the modern era, that status has been maintained and possibly expanded, with contemporary teachers all emphasising the importance of Patañjali's work, and new translations appearing with quite startling regularity. In the 1990s, Barbara Stoler Miller produced a new translation and commentary, which is highly recommended, in 2001 T.S. Rukmani provided a valuable edition that includes a translation of Vyasa's commentary, and as recently as 2008 a new Penguin Classics edition appeared in which Shyam Ranganathan sought to demonstrate that Patañjali's primary concern was with moral philosophy.

ENGLISH TRANSLATIONS OF THE YOGA SŪTRAS

One of the main problems confronting anyone seeking to get an insight into the teachings of the *Yoga Sūtras* is that English translations vary so dramatically from one another, to the extent where it can be very difficult to properly determine exactly what Patañjali does and does not say. There will, of course, always be differences in translations of any work, as different translators see different meanings, and in some cases bring their own preconceptions to bear. This is certainly true of some English editions of the *Yoga Sūtras*, such as the Penguin Classics version in which Shyam Ranganathan holds to a rather unusual reading. Beyond these issues, however, there are particular difficulties involved with Patañjali's writing due to the highly technical vocabulary he employs, and the extremely dense *sūtra* style adopted. It seems certain that this and other similar works were composed in *sūtras* so that the meaning could be conveyed in the fewest words possible, and the whole of the text could be more easily committed to memory. In the *Yoga Sūtras*, we find that virtually no verbs are employed, and it is left to the reader to fill in the implicit meaning, which is deemed to be self-evident. The problem is of course that to the modern reader the meaning is often by no means self-evident, and the teaching of particular passages is therefore rendered obscure.

The translation included here is original, but must be regarded as just one amongst many, and by no means a definitive version. As far as possible I have tried to preserve the original sense of the text without imposition of meaning, but it is often necessary to unpack the language in order to convey the intended sense of the words; if words were to be omitted, as they are in the Sanskrit, then in many cases the English translation would be without meaning. I have also tended to leave much of the technical language untranslated, partly because there are very often no real equivalents in English, and partly because the text itself frequently presents a word or idea, and then proceeds to explain what this means. In such circumstances, there seems little point in using an English approximation that can never fully capture the true sense of the Sanskrit original.

THE STRUCTURE AND CONTENT OF THE YOGA SŪTRAS

There are four chapters or sections to our text, which are named respectively as the *Samādhi-pāda*, the *Sādhana-pāda*, the *Vibhūti-pāda*, and the *Kaivalya-pāda*, with the title of each section being broadly approximate to the content. Each of the first three parts is of almost the same length, including 51, 55 and 56 *sūtras* respectively. The *Kaivalya-pāda* is a little shorter with only 34 *sūtras*, yielding a total of 196 *sūtras* for the entire work.

It must be recognised that in spite of the title, Patañjali did not set out to compile a manual of Yoga practice that the aspirant could take home and use for him or herself. There is in fact very little to be found within the *sūtras* that can be regarded as direct instruction as to how the aspiring *yogin* should conduct himself in order to achieve the designated goals. Rather the *Yoga Sūtras* should properly be seen as a text delineating the philosophy of Yoga, explaining why it is necessary, what it can achieve, how it can be efficacious, and the type of practice that is to be undertaken. There is, however, a big distinction to be drawn between outlining the type of practice and giving step by step directions as to how this is to be undertaken. Patañjali certainly completes the former of these tasks, but seems to leave the latter to the teachers who will lead their followers through the minutiae of daily ritual. And this factor in turn has allowed teachers of different types of Yoga to refer to Patañjali as their basic authority, even where the practices they advocate have very little to do with the explicit content of the *Yoga Sūtras*.

Broadly speaking, it does seem that Patañjali accepts the fundamental premises of the Sāṁkhya view of the world. Essentially, the *puruṣa*, or true self, is entangled within the domain of matter, and as a result of this entanglement it must experience misery and misfortune. The root cause of this situation is ignorance, *avidyā*, which covers the *puruṣa*, and conceals its own true identity. In place of the truth, it identifies instead with external movements of the mind, as it roams through the world gathering up mental impressions, which then become attached to the *puruṣa*, and carry it forward as it transmigrates from body to body. Patañjali therefore advocates the suspension of this external mental focus, so that the impressions gathered cease to attach themselves to the *puruṣa*, and the veil of *avidyā* can be lifted through intense introspective activity.

This might be called the philosophy of Yoga, its raison d'etre, which is set out in the opening *Samādhi-pāda*. The *Sādhana-pāda* then provides us with more details of the actual practice to be undertaken, and it is here that we encounter the notion of the eight limbs, *aṣṭa aṅga*, of Yoga. The first five of these are delineated in the second chapter, but these are declared to be external or preparatory to the final flowering of the practice, which is achieved through the final three limbs, collectively designated as the *saṁyama*. It is the discussion of *saṁyama* that forms the main theme of the opening section of the *Vibhūti-pāda*, and this in turn leads into a consideration of the wondrous results that can be achieved through the diligent practice of *aṣṭāṅga-yoga*.

These results are of two differing types. Firstly, magical and supernatural powers arise, so that the adept is able to transcend the laws of nature by flying through the air, or reading the minds of others. Above and beyond such amazing feats, however, the *yogin* can also achieve the highest spiritual goal, which, as in the Sāṁkhya *darśana*, is defined as *kaivalya*, literally the separation of the *puruṣa* from its entanglement with matter, the latter referred to by the term *prakṛti*, or occasionally *pradhāna*. It is this idea of *mokṣa*, liberation from the cycle of rebirth, which is presented as the ultimate goal of Yoga practice, and which forms the main subject for discussion in the fourth and final section. And in this we can see what Yoga actually was in this early period, namely the techniques through which the adept could attain the level of realisation required for the soul to break free of its bondage in matter.

THE WIDER CONTEXT OF THE YOGA SŪTRAS

In the earlier discussion of the dating of the *Yoga Sūtras*, it was suggested that this work is very probably later than the *Mahābhārata*'s Yoga treatises, and the *Bhagavad-gītā*, and may very well have made use of these earlier works on Yoga. Whether or not this was the case, it is clear that the type of Yoga practice advocated within the *Yoga Sūtras* is broadly equivalent to that advocated in these two texts. It is this form of practice that is commonly referred to as 'classical Yoga' as a way of contrasting it with the Tantric or Haṭha Yoga more commonly encountered in the modern era. We should, moreover, be aware of the significant Buddhist and Jain influence on Indian thought during the period when the *Yoga Sūtras* was compiled, and it is certainly possible to identify ideas and terminology that Patañjali shares with these other traditions.

What becomes readily apparent as we read through the *Yoga Sūtras* is that this text is closely integrated into the wider context of Indian religious thought, and the central theme of gaining liberation from rebirth. This imperative towards *mokṣa* is shared with the Sāṁkhya and Vedānta systems, with the Jain and Buddhist traditions, and with most of the devotional expressions of Hinduism as well. Hence it is important to see Patañjali's revelations in this light in order to understand his primary intention in compiling the *Yoga Sūtras*. As the Buddha taught, life is primarily characterised by suffering, as each being progresses through an endless cycle of rebirth. Yoga philosophy teaches the process through which rebirth is perpetuated, as each action and each thought leaves a latent impression on the consciousness, which must at some point come to fruition as material existence is carried forward. What Patañjali is offering here is not just an explanation of the process, but also a concomitant means of ending it. If the activity of the mind can be stilled in some way, then the creation of new impressions will also cease, and these in turn will then cease to generate further rebirths. The Yoga system is proposed as a means by which the action of the mind can be stilled, and the progression of rebirth finally concluded thereby.

With these thoughts in mind, let us now proceed to study each of the four *pādas* in turn so that we can acquire a greater insight into the explanation of life in this world, the process of cessation, and goals to be achieved.

CHAPTER 1: THE SAMĀDHI-PĀDA

THIS first section of the *Yoga Sūtras* provides an explanation of what Yoga is, and what its aims are. Patañjali's usual style is to introduce a concept briefly, and then build upon it in the ensuing *sūtras*, so that it is hard to understand a single *sūtra* when taken out of context. The text thus builds progressively, and it is important to follow the pattern, as it is clear that the overall structure is carefully designed. We will bear these points in mind as we begin our reading.

1–4: THE PURPOSE OF YOGA

1. *atha yogānuśāsanam,*
   Here is the teaching on Yoga.

2. *yogaś citta-vṛtti-nirodhaḥ,*
   Yoga is the restriction of the movements of the mind.

3. *tadā draṣṭuḥ sva-rūpe 'vasthānam,*
   When this is achieved, the witness comes to exist in terms of its true identity.

4. *vṛtti-sārūpyam itiratra,*
   Otherwise, the witness assumes the identity dictated by the movement of the mind.

This opening passage is vitally important for understanding

the *Yoga Sūtras* as a whole. The first *sūtra* simply acts as an introduction, but in *sūtra* 2, we have the definition of Yoga on which the entire work is based: *citta-vṛtti-nirodha.* The use of the word *citta* is a little unusual, as it does not appear in the usual Sāṁkhya analyses of the human consciousness. Sāṁkhya typically speaks of *manas*, *buddhi* and *ahaṁkāra*, mind, intellect, and a sense of self, as jointly comprising the mental faculty, and so we must consider what is meant here by the word *citta*, as it is a term that Patañjali uses repeatedly.

Barbara Stoler Miller insists that it should be understood as 'thoughts', but this tends to give an impression of something the mind does rather than being integral to the person. It would probably be better to understand *citta* as the thinking faculty, and in fact most translators opt for 'mind', which is probably as close as we can get in English. The word *vṛtti* means movement or activity, and hence *citta-vṛtti* means the different types of mental activity the thought process pursues. And *nirodha* means to restrict or to inhibit, so *citta-vṛtti-nirodha* means to inhibit the fluctuations of the mind as it follows its conventional patterns of thought. Hence we should note from the outset that the type of Yoga Patañjali is delineating is a Yoga of the mind rather than of the body.

The third *sūtra* then reveals the purpose behind this Yoga practice, namely to allow the *draṣṭṛ* to remain in its true form. The word *draṣṭṛ* literally means one who observes, and here we must regard it as referring to the *puruṣa* or *ātman*, the true self that exists in a state beyond matter. Hence its natural *sva-rūpa*, or true form, is to be untouched by the limitations we must endure in life; it is this state of liberation that Yoga is designed to bring about, freeing the soul from its unnatural condition of embodiment.

Sūtra 4 then tells us more about the alternative state of existence for the *draṣṭṛ*, a false condition in which it loses contact with its true identity, and instead assumes the condition imposed upon it by the *vṛtti*, the fluctuations of the mind. Essentially what Patañjali is saying here is that the identity we conceive for ourselves is not a true identity, it is simply a reflection of our state of mind. If the *vṛttis* can be curtailed, then the false material identities they impose upon the soul will cease to exist, and the soul will return to its natural state beyond the miseries of this existence. This then establishes what Yoga is about, what it consists of, and what it is designed to achieve.

5–12: CITTA–VṚTTI DEFINED

5. *vṛttayaḥ pañcatayyaḥ kliṣṭākliṣṭāḥ,*
   The movements of the mind can be divided into five categories; these can either bring affliction or be free of affliction.

6. *pramāṇa-viparyaya-vikalpa-nidrā-smṛtayaḥ,*
   These five are proper judgement, false assessment, uncertainty, sleep, and the remembrance of things past.

7. *pratyakṣānumānāgamāḥ pramāṇāni,*
   Proper judgement comes from direct perception, logical inference, and scriptural revelation.

8. *viparyayo mithyā-jñānam atad-rūpa-pratiṣṭham,*
   False assessment means misunderstanding based on mistaken apprehension of the object.

9. *śabda-jñānānupātī vastu-śūnyo vikalpaḥ,*
   Uncertainty arises when knowledge is based on words alone, and is devoid of a proper object of perception.

10. *abhāva-pratyayālambanā vṛttir nidrā,*
    Sleep is where the movement of the mind has no object on which to focus.

11. *anubhūta-viṣayāsaṃpramoṣaḥ smṛtiḥ,*
Remembrance is where the experience of an object is retained.

These *sūtras* seek to expand on the idea of *citta-vṛtti*, introduced in the second *sūtra*. What are these fluctuations or movements of our thought processes? We now learn that they can be categorised firstly as twofold, and then into five categories. The twofold division is as *kliṣṭa* and *akliṣṭa*, causing pain or being troublesome, and then not causing affliction. *Sūtra* 6 lists the five types of *citta-vṛtti*, but it is not made clear whether it is two, three, or four of the five that are *kliṣṭa*, and the remainder *akliṣṭa*, or whether all five can be sometimes troublesome and sometimes benign; the latter seems to be more likely.

The five types of *citta-vṛtti* are listed as *pramāṇa*, reaching a proper judgement, *viparyaya*, false understanding of a situation, *vikalpa*, not being able to reach any certainty, *nidrā*, sleep, and *smṛti*, memory or recollection. As we have seen, Yoga is defined as the process by which these five mental activities are brought to an end. Five *sūtras*, 7 to 11, then describe each of the *citta-vṛttis* in turn. *Pramāṇa*, proper understanding, can be gained from direct perception, from inference, and from the revelation of the *āgamas*, or sacred texts. This idea of how true knowledge is acquired is one that is shared with other *darṣanas*, including the Sāṁkhya and Vedānta systems. *Viparyaya*, wrong understanding, is the exact opposite of *pramāṇa*; it is not derived from any of the three solid bases of knowledge, but rather rests upon *mithyā*-jñāna, false or wrong knowledge of what something truly is. *Vikalpa* is the state where one cannot determine between *pramāṇa* and *viparyaya*, and is left in a condition of uncertainty.

The final two *vṛttis* are *nidrā* and *smṛti*, sleep and memory. Here it seems that *nidrā* indicates the state of deep dreamless sleep referred to in the *Māṇḍūkya Upaniṣad* (5). In this state, the mind has no tangible object on which to focus, and yet it cannot be said to be wholly inactive. Therefore this condition is also included amongst the movements of the mind. *Smṛti* is the process whereby the sensory encounter with a particular object is not lost, so that the flavour, smell, sight, or feel of the object can be recalled and recognised at a later date.

These then are the *citta-vṛttis* that must be brought to a state of *nirodha* through the practice of Yoga.

12–16: THE MEANING OF NIRODHA

12. *abhyāsa-vairāgyābhyāṁ tan-nirodhaḥ,*
The restriction of these movements of the mind is achieved through regular practice, and through renunciation.

13. *tatra sthitau yatno 'bhyāsaḥ,*
Regular practice means the exertion required to achieve steadiness of the mind.

14. *sa tu dīrgha-kāla-nairantarya-satkārāsevito dṛḍha-bhūmiḥ,*
Now when this exertion is properly performed for a long time, without interruption, it becomes firmly established.

15. *dṛṣṭānu śravika-viṣaya-vitṛṣṇasya vaśīkāra-saṁjñā vairāgyam,*
Renunciation is known to be the self-mastery that removes the hankering arising from perceiving or learning about an object.

16. *tat-paraṁ puruṣa-khyāter guṇa-vaitṛṣṇyam,*
A superior form of renunciation is the lack of hankering for material attributes that arises from realisation of the *puruṣa*, the true self.

In this next passage the meaning is provided for another of the terms used in the definition of Yoga found in *sūtra* 2. *Nirodha* means the restriction or the cessation of the *citta-vṛttis* previously discussed. First we are told how this is to be accomplished; it is through *abhyāsa* and *vairāgya*, exactly the same terms as are used by Kṛṣṇa in the *Bhagavad-gītā* when he rejects Arjuna's complaint that Yoga is virtually impossible (6.35). It is difficult, but *nirodha* can certainly be achieved through continual practice, *abhyāsa*, and by turning away from worldly aspirations, *vairāgya*. *Sūtras* 13 and 14 then further define *abhyāsa*, whilst 15 and 16 explain how *vairāgya* is to be accomplished. The practice of Yoga must be resolute and sustained if it is to be successful, and must be carried on uninterruptedly over a long period of time. Only dedication of this type will bring success.

Vairāgya can be achieved by overcoming the longing we feel when the senses perceive a desirable object. This clearly requires a great effort of will, but in *sūtra* 16 a superior form of *vairāgya* is noted, whereby detachment from the material world is achieved through realisation of the spiritual entity, the *puruṣa*, that is the true self. Here again, I think, we can note a link to the *Bhagavad-gītā* (2.59) in which full detachment from this world is said to be achieved by perceiving the spiritual joy that comes through realisation of the higher domain, *paraṁ dṛṣṭvā nivartate*. These *sūtras* thus explain that the *nirodha* mentioned in *sūtra* 2 can be achieved only by constant and resolute practice, and by detaching oneself from the world either by an effort of will, or better still by realisation of the spiritual truth that abides within one's own being as the *puruṣa*.

17–20: SAṂPRAJÑĀTA AND ASAṂPRAJÑĀTA REALISATION

17. *vitarka-vicārānandāsmitā-*
rūpānugamāt saṁprajñātaḥ,

Where this realisation is conscious, it is achieved through deliberation, reflection, joy, and the experience of selfhood.

18. *virāma-pratyayābhyāsa-pūrvaḥ saṃskāra-śeṣo 'nyaḥ,*
The other type of realisation is preceded by the practice of suppressing conscious thought so that only subconscious impressions remain.

19. *bhava-pratyayo videha-prakṛti-layānām,*
For beings who do not have bodies, and whose physical forms have merged back into *prakṛti*, mental processes focus on existence alone.

20. *śraddhā-vīrya-smṛti-samādhi-prajñā-pūrvaka itareṣām,*
Others attain this state preceded by faith, vigorous endeavour, recollection, *samādhi*, and realised knowledge.

Here one must presume that Patañjali is expanding upon the idea of *puruṣa-khyāti*, realisation of the *puruṣa*, introduced in *sūtra* 16. We are now told that this realisation can be of two kinds, with and without conscious thoughts, designated as *saṁprajñāta* and *anya*, meaning the other or the opposite, which we may therefore take as *asaṁprajñāta*. As always, when states of consciousness are being discussed it is difficult for one who is not an expert in Yoga practice to determine exactly what is meant by the discussion. *Saṁprajñāta* realisation is said to be based on *vitarka, vicāra, ānanda* and *asmita*, conscious deliberation, reflection, a sense of joy, and an awareness of oneself. This would seem to indicate that this type of realisation is based on reflective insight, by which one tries to make sense of one's own identity, and reaches the conclusion that there must be a soul that is above and beyond the overt personality.

Asaṁprajñāta realisation, by contrast, occurs when such conscious reason is suppressed, and is replaced by an unchanging awareness of the *puruṣa* that is not dependent on thought or reason. For most persons, this type of higher realised consciousness, which transcends the thought processes, is simply a theoretical concept, but it is towards this state that the process of *citta-vṛtti-nirodha* is aspiring. *Saṁprajñāta* realisation seems to be based on reasoned conviction whilst the other type of realisation is experiential. And because it is not dependent on reason or mental activity, it can also be sustained by beings who do not possess bodies, which according to Vyasa refers to the gods, or beings who live in higher worlds. For such higher beings, *asaṁprajñāta* realisation is natural, but for others it can be attained through a variety of means including faith, endeavour, recollection, *samādhi*, and knowledge.

We must recall again that these two types of realisation were related to the higher path of *citta-vṛtti-nirodha* where *nirodha* is achieved by realisation of the true self. We now have two means by which this realisation of the self is achieved, one by conscious thought processes, and the other by transcending such processes.

21–22: THE NECESSITY OF ENDEAVOUR

21. *tīvra-saṃvegānām āsannaḥ*
This state is very near for those who display ardent intensity in their practice.

22. *mṛdu-madhyādhimātratvāt tato 'pi viśeṣaḥ*
As persons are leisurely, middling, or intense in their practice, so excellence is achieved accordingly.

These two *sūtras* seem relatively straightforward and can be regarded as referring back to *sūtras* 12 and 13, in which *abhyāsa*, regular practice, was given as one of the means by which *citta-vṛtti-nirodha* can be achieved. Now we are told that when the *abhyāsa* is intense or committed, realisation will be close, but if it is only middling or mild then the level of realisation will be commensurate. In other words, success in Yoga practice is dependent on the amount of dedication one is willing to give to it.

23–28: DEVOTION TO ĪŚVARA

23. *īśvara-praṇidhānād vā,*
Or it may be achieved by devoting oneself to the Lord.

24. *kleśa-karma-vipākāśayair aparāmṛṣṭaḥ puruṣa-viśeṣa īśvaraḥ,*
Īśvara (the Deity or Lord) is a special *puruṣa*, free from the influence of affliction, action, the ripening of accumulated *karma*, or latent impressions.

25. *tatra niratiśayaṃ sarva-jñatva-bījam,*
For the *īśvara*, the seed of omniscience has grown to a state that cannot be surpassed.

26. *sa pūrveṣām api guruḥ kālenānavacchedāt,*
He was also the *guru* of the ancient teachers, for he is unrestricted by time.

27. *tasya vācakaḥ praṇavaḥ,*
His sound form is *praṇava, oṃkāra.*

28. *taj-japas-tad-artha-bhāvanam,*
The quiet repetition (*japa*) of that sound makes its object become manifest.

It has to be admitted that ideas of this type are rather unusual within the context of Yoga discourse, and my suspicion is that they reflect Patañjali's awareness of, and respect for, the teachings of the *Bhagavad-gītā*, which is overtly theistic. It is also the case, however, that passages on Yoga within the *Mahābhārata* include the assertion that it is reverence for a Supreme Deity that distinguishes the adherents of the Yoga system from the followers of Sāṁkhya.

Here the word *vā* in *sūtra* 23 indicates that *īśvara-praṇidhāna* is another means by which realisation can be attained, in addition to the *saṁprajñāta* and *asaṁprajñāta* just considered. The word *īśvara* is frequently used in Hindu religious literature to refer to the Supreme Deity of monotheistic doctrines, whilst *praṇidhāna* can mean either veneration for, or intense focus upon, a particular object. In this context, veneration would seem to be the more natural meaning.

Sūtras 24 to 27, however, then define *īśvara* in a manner that must raise questions as to the extent to which Patañjali is truly expounding the type of monotheistic teaching found within the *Bhagavad-gītā*, and most notably in the writings of medieval *ācāryas* such as Rāmānuja and Madhva. *Sūtra* 24 declares that the *īśvara* is a *viśeṣa puruṣa*, a special or superior soul, a term that might be taken as equivalent to *puruṣa uttama* or *puruṣottama*, which the *Gītā* uses to refer to the Deity in its fifteenth chapter. Why is this *puruṣa* different from all others? It is because he is beyond all affliction, and is untouched by the influence of karma, and because the 'seed of omniscience' has reached full fruition.

These explanations are interesting because they could perfectly well be applied to any *puruṣa* that has achieved *kaivalya*, the state of liberation in which *puruṣa* separates itself entirely from matter. If the *īśvara* is simply a liberated *puruṣa* then the claim that the *Yoga Sūtras* is theistic in orientation must be seriously called into question. It is also noteworthy that at no point does Patañjali take up the *Bhagavad-gītā*'s idea that liberation can be acquired as a gift of grace from a loving God. At all times, *kaivalya* is presented as a goal to be achieved by personal endeavour, by *abhyāsa* and *vairāgya*, and not by *deva-prasāda*, the grace of God.

I think *sūtra* 26 is particularly interesting in its assertion that *īśvara* is the *guru* of those who appeared in ancient times, and who is not restricted by time, as this seems to be directly related to the opening verses of Chapter 4 of the *Gītā*, and may well be derived from them. There Kṛṣṇa states that he originally taught Yoga to the sun god, Vivasvān, *imaṁ vivasvate yogaṁ proktavān aham*, and when Arjuna questions how this is possible, Kṛṣṇa replies that he appears many times, uninhibited by the influence of time.

We are then told that the syllable *om* is the Deity's *vācaka*, the sound that represents him, and that he becomes manifest to one who resonates this sound. *Om* or *praṇava* is referred to on a number of occasions in the *Upaniṣads* as the sound that is equivalent to Brahman, the supreme principle, and in the *Māṇḍūkya Upaniṣad* it is declared that all things are simply *om*, *sarvam oṁkāra eva* (1). The *Yoga Sūtras* does not fully expand upon its understanding of the nature of *īśvara*, and hence there must be some doubt about the extent of its theistic tendencies; we should, however, be cautious about presuming that Patañjali advocates a notion of God that can be accepted as consonant with Western or Indian monotheisms, or indeed the monistic ideas advocated by the Advaita school of Vedānta.

29–32: OBSTACLES TO PROGRESS

29. *tataḥ pratyak-cetanādhigamo 'py antarāyābhāvaś ca,*
At that point one achieves the state of inward contemplation, and the obstacles to practice cease to exist.

30. *vyādhi-styāna-saṁśaya-ramādālasyāvirati-bhrānti-darśanālabdha-bhūmikatvānavasthitatvāni citta-vikṣepās te 'ntarāyāḥ,*

These obstacles that distract the mind are disease, sloth, doubt, negligence, indolence, indulgence, misapprehension, failure to keep one's understanding firmly grounded, and a lack of consistency in one's practice.

31. *duḥkha-daurmanasyāṅgam-ejayatva-śvāsa-praśvāsā vikṣepa-sahabhuvaḥ,*
The distractions are accompanied by distress, dejection, trembling of the body, and heavy inward and outward breathing.

32. *tat-pratiṣedhārtham eka-tattvābhyāsaḥ,*
In order to overcome the obstacles, one should engage in regular practice aimed at a single object.

These *sūtras* are concerned with the obstacles to Yoga, and how they may be overcome. The word *tataḥ* in *sūtra* 29 literally means 'from that', and therefore must logically refer to the *japa* of *om* mentioned in 28. The result of this *japa* is twofold, firstly the mind is directed inwards away from external perception through the senses, and secondly the obstacles to progress cease to exist. *Sūtra* 30 lists the obstacles and describes their effect on the *yogin* as *citta-vikṣepa*, which means that they scatter the movements of the mind in all directions. As the aim of Yoga is to suppress the movements of the mind, it is logical to see that the obstacles should have the opposite effect. In 31, it is stated that as the distractions become predominant, one feels a sense of distress and frustration, and then in 32 we are told that the distractions can be overcome only by single-minded *abhyāsa*, in other words by dedication to the task, and making it the topmost goal. The next verses then build on this more hopeful assertion by discussing *citta-prasāda*, serenity of mind, which one presumes is the opposite of *citta-vikṣepa*, distraction of the mind as it scatters in all directions.

33–40: SERENITY OF MIND AND HOW TO ACHIEVE IT

33. *maitrī-karuṇā-muditopekṣāṇāṁ sukha-duḥkha-puṇyāpuṇya-viṣayāṇāṁ bhāvanātaś citta-prasādanam,*
Serenity of mind is achieved when one shows friendship towards those who are happy, compassion for those who suffer, delight towards the righteous, and indifference towards the wicked.

34. *pracchardana-vidhāraṇābhyāṁ vā prāṇasya,*
Such serenity may also be achieved through the exhaling and the retention of the breath.

35. *viṣayavatī vā pravṛttir-utpannā manasaḥ sthiti-nibandhinī,*
Or by controlling the mind, and making it still when it becomes active in relation to an object.

36. *viṣokā vā jyotiṣmatī,*
Or by remaining free of sorrow, and filled with light.

37. *vīta-rāga-viṣayaṁ vā cittam,*
Or when the mind is free of longing for any object.

38. *svapna-nidrā-jñānālambanaṁ vā,*
Or by focusing upon the realisation acquired whilst dreaming, or in a state of deep sleep.

39. *yathābhimata-dhyānād vā,*
Or by meditating on any object one likes.

40. *paramāṇu-parama-mahattvānto 'sya vaśīkāraḥ,*
The result of this mental serenity is that one gains control over that which is the most minute, and that which is the largest thing.

The *sūtras* in this passage expand upon the phrase *eka-tattvābhyāsa*, single-minded practice, from *sūtra* 32, by explaining different ways in which this practice can be undertaken. The result of this *abhyāsa* is *citta-prasāda*, which can be taken as the antithesis of the *citta-vikṣepa* that the obstacles produce. I am not sure, however, that we should take *citta-prasāda* to be equivalent to *citta-vṛtti-nirodha*, which is the goal of Yoga practice, and it is probably better to regard it as a state of mind conducive to progress in Yoga, devoid of the obstacles discussed above. This view would seem to be confirmed by the different ways through which this serenity of mind can be achieved, which do not involve the full eightfold practice that will be outlined in the *Sādhana-pāda*, the second chapter of the *Yoga Sūtras*.

The methods for achieving this positive outlook and serene state of mind begin from *sūtra* 33, which describes the appropriate manner of relating to persons of different types. One should be joyful when others find happiness, feel compassion for those who suffer, take delight in other people's virtue, and feel indifference, rather than hostility, towards wicked-minded persons. Then other more technical methods are presented. Firstly, there is breath control, then holding back the mind from its preoccupation with external objects, then refusing to indulge excessively in grief or regret, and then limiting the extent of material desires. *Sūtra* 38 refers to the belief that insight or realisations can enter the unconscious mind whilst a person is in a state of sleep, and that truth can be revealed through dreams. Hence it is stated here that paying close attention to these subconscious revelations is another means by which *citta-prasāda* is gained. And the final method, given in *sūtra* 39, is *dhyāna yathā abhimata*, meditation on a particular object one is drawn towards. Here one presumes that the fact that the object is one of choice makes meditation upon it easier to achieve, and the goal is to limit the *citta-vikṣepa*, the scattering of the mind, so that *citta-prasāda* emerges in its place. In the final *sūtra* of this passage (40), we get an indication that one who achieves such serenity of mind obtains an inner strength that allows mastery over great and small things. This may be a reference to the supernatural powers described in Chapter 3 of the *Yoga Sūtras*, or it may simply mean that a person who achieves such serenity has the mental strength that brings success in all endeavours.

41–46: THE STATE OF SAMĀPATTI

41. *kṣīṇa-vṛtter abhijātasyeva maṇer grahītṛ-grahaṇa-grāhyeṣu tat-stha-tad-añjanatā samāpattiḥ,*
When the movements of the mind are weakened, it becomes like a clear gemstone, assuming the form of the perceiver, the process of perception, and the object of perception. This state of absorption of the mind is called *samāpatti.*

42. *tatra śabdārtha-jñāna-vikalpaiḥ saṁkīrṇā sa-vitarkā samāpattiḥ,*
Where this state is adulterated by uncertainty in understanding words and their meaning, it is to be known as *samāpatti* mixed with conscious deliberation.

43. *smṛti-pariśuddhau svarūpa-śūnyevārtha-mātra-nirbhāsā nirvitarkā,*
But when the memory is purified, the external form of the object disappears and it shines forth alone. This state is called *samāpatti* free of conscious deliberation.

44. *etayaiva sa-vicārā nirvicārā ca sūkṣma-viṣayā vyākhyātā,*
In this way, *samāpatti* focused on subtle objects, with and without reflective modes of thought, has now been explained.

45. *sūkṣma-viṣayatvam cāliṅga-paryavasānam,*
As has the subtle nature of objects which occurs when external characteristics are no longer present.

46. *tā eva sa-bījaḥ samādhiḥ,*
These practices, defined as *samāpatti,* are to be known as *samādhi* arising from a seed.

In this passage we are taken back to the earlier line of discussion that is more directly related to the topic of the chapter as a whole, namely *citta-vṛtti-nirodha,* the stilling of the movements of the mind, which is what Yoga amounts to. Here a new concept, *samāpatti,* is introduced and defined in relation to the wider process. The term *samāpatti* is often taken as being equivalent to *samādhi,* the ultimate state of consciousness that Yoga is striving towards, but here I think we can see that this equation is only partially valid; in fact *samāpatti* is the preliminary stage of *samādhi,* and not the full state of absolute realisation. The word *samāpatti* is derived from the verb *sam-ā-pad,* which means to attain or enter a particular place or condition, and hence a loose translation might be 'realisation', but there seems little point in using any term other than the original Sanskrit word.

Sūtra 41 gives an explanation of what is meant by *samāpatti,* although as always it is difficult to say precisely what this state of consciousness amounts to. *Samāpatti* occurs when previous practice has brought success by reducing the *citta-vṛttis,* the movements of the mind. In the previous mental condition, there is a clear distinction between the perceiver, the object, and the process of perception, but Yoga practice now brings about a state of intense clarity in which those distinctions are removed, as the mind becomes utterly still. Of course, this verbal explanation cannot come close to replicating the experience Patañjali is referring to, but for now it must suffice.

Sūtras 42 and 43 provide further elaboration by revealing

that the state of *samāpatti* is twofold, defined as *sa-vitarka* and *nir-vitarka*, with and without *vitarka*. We have encountered a rather similar idea earlier in the chapter in relation to *saṁprajñāta* and *asaṁprajñāta* realisation (*sūtras* 17-20), although we must not necessarily presume that it is exactly the same concept being considered here. What does seem to be apparent is that *samāpatti* can be achieved whilst the conscious mind is still active in some way, *sa-vitarkā samāpatti*, and then when conscious deliberation is wholly stilled as *nir-vitarkā samāpatti*. As far as can be understood, *sa-vitarkā samāpatti* is a state in which the mind is consciously focused on the characteristics of an object and *nir-vitarkā samāpatti* is where the mind is wholly absorbed in contemplating the object, but without any conscious thoughts relating to it.

Sūtras 44 and 45 conclude by stating that this account has covered *sa-vicāra*, *nir-vicāra* and *sūkṣma-viṣaya*. As we have seen, there is not a great deal of difference between *vicāra* and *vitarka*, and it is probably the case that here Patañjali is pointing out that *sa-* and *nir-vitarkā samāpatti* are also *sa-vicāra* and *nir-vicāra*. *Sūkṣma-viṣaya* means subtle objects, and I take this to mean the nature of an object when the mind is absorbed in consciousness of it without reflective thought. Here the mind is not fixed on the qualities and features of the object, after the manner of conscious thought, but is simply absorbed in its absolute nature, and it is this that is being referred to as the subtle nature of the object, transcending the overt qualities that are the subject of conscious reflection. And in *sūtra* 46, we are informed that *samāpatti* is equivalent to *samādhi*, but only *sa-bīja samādhi*, *samādhi* with a seed, presumably because even where the *samāpatti* is *nir-vitarka* there is still an object involved, at least in a seed form.

47–51: THE NATURE OF NIRBĪJA SAMĀDHI

47. nirvicāra-vaiśāradye 'dhyātma-prasādaḥ,
When one attains perfection in *samāpatti* free of conscious reflection, one gains a serenity directly related to the *ātman*, the soul.

48. ṛtambharā tatra prajñā,
The realisation acquired in this way is laden with *ṛta*, absolute truth.

49. śrutānumāna-prajñābhyām anya-viṣayā viśeṣārthavāt,
This realisation has a different object to that acquired through the scriptures or through inference, because it is directed towards a higher purpose.

50. taj-jaḥ saṁskāro 'nya-saṁskāra-pratibandhī,
The latent impression on the mind generated by this realisation serves to neutralise other latent impressions.

51. tasyāpi nirodhe sarva-nirodhān nirbījaḥ samādhiḥ,
When even that movement of the mind is also restricted, all movements are restricted, and the state known as seedless *samādhi* is then achieved.

In this final passage of the *Samādhi-pāda*, we reach the ultimate conclusion of this section of the discourse, as Patañjali reveals the final stage of Yoga realisation, which he defines in *sūtra* 51 as *nirbīja samādhi*, seedless *samādhi*. Further insight is provided by *sūtra* 47, which informs us that this ultimate attainment comes when one achieves perfection in the *nir-vicārā samāpatti* previously discussed; and it is also defined there as *adhyātma-prasāda*. We encountered the word *prasāda* a few *sutras* earlier where *citta-prasāda*, serenity of mind, was presented as an alternative to *citta-vikṣepa*, scattering of the mental processes. The word *adhyātma* is found in the *Bhagavad-gītā* and *Upaniṣads*, but probably more significantly within the *Mahābhārata*'s discourses on Sāṁkhya where knowledge of the *ātman*, the true self, is designated as the science of *adhyātma*. Here then I think we can presume that *adhyātma-prasāda* means the absolute serenity that is gained through realisation of the *ātman*. *Nir-bīja-samādhi* is thus to be equated with realisation of the true self, the spiritual entity that is the true essence of our being.

Sūtra 48 states that the knowledge attained in this way is *ṛta-ambhara*, or saturated with *ṛta*. The word *ṛta* is found in the earliest Vedic texts where it is often taken as broadly equivalent to dharma, meaning the proper order of things. Here the knowledge acquired through Yoga is described as being *ṛta*, imbued with the highest level of truth, in other words the truth of the soul's spiritual identity.

This point is clarified in 49 and 50, which assert that this knowledge is superior even to that gained from scripture (because it has a different object), and that the impressions it generates overwhelm all the other impressions that shape and reshape the mind. Here we may recall the statement of *sūtra* 7, which gave the three sources of knowledge as *pratyakṣa* (perception), *anumāna* (inference), and *āgama* (scripture). Here we must take *śruta* as being equivalent to *āgama*, which leads us to the conclusion that the realisation gained through Yoga is based on direct perception. In other words, Yoga practice brings the practitioner inward perception that ultimately allows for experiential knowledge of the spiritual reality to develop. Like all perceptions, this too creates a *saṁskāra*, a latent impression upon the mind, and this *saṁskāra* drives away all the material impressions that produce ignorance and rebirth. And finally this *saṁskāra* is also removed so that the soul exists in its true identity, as was asserted at the beginning in *sūtras* 3 and 4. Here again there is an alignment of ideas with the teachings of the *Bhagavad-gītā*, as in both works we find the teaching that the culmination of Yoga practice is realisation of spiritual wisdom based on direct perception of the true self.

CHAPTER 2: THE SĀDHANA-PĀDA

THE second chapter of the *Yoga Sūtras* is entitled the *Sādhana-Pada*. The word *sādhana* comes from the verb *sadh*, which literally means to travel straight towards a goal, and hence, as you might expect, *sādhana* indicates the proper means to achieve the goal. The term is still commonly employed in contemporary Hinduism to indicate the regulated practices or rituals undertaken in religious life.

Hence whilst the first chapter focused primarily on mental states, and the stilling of the mind, this second section deals with the practical steps by which this is achieved, and thereby introduces the eight limbs of Yoga. Before we get directly on to the *sādhana*, however, there are extensive preliminaries to go through, and the chapter is probably best understood as falling into three units of discourse.

The opening section, including *sūtras* 1 to 17, deals primarily with the problem of human existence, which is analysed in terms somewhat similar to Buddhist teaching. As the Buddha taught in his first noble truth, life according to Patañjali is predominated by affliction and suffering, which arises as karmic reactions come to fruition. This then is the problem faced by all human beings, but in the second section of the chapter (*sūtras* 18 to 27), it is revealed that the problem can be resolved, and that in fact the material manifestation exists solely for the purpose of enabling the soul to liberate itself from affliction, a view that is also to be found in Ishvara Krishna's *Sāṁkhya Kārikā*. Once these two preliminary points have been made, the second half of the chapter is given over to directly addressing the issue of *sādhana*. Here the eight limbs of Yoga are listed, and then the first five of these are discussed in more detail, with most attention being paid to the first two of the limbs, *yama* and *niryama*.

One might be tempted to suggest that a direct Buddhist influence can be detected in the division of the chapter into these three areas of discussion. These can certainly be equated with three of Buddha's four noble truths, although the fact that there are eight limbs of Yoga and an eightfold path prescribed by the Buddha is almost certainly coincidental. It is also the case that at the time when the *Yoga Sūtras* was probably composed Buddhist thought had a position of great significance in Indian religion, but I would be reluctant to press the notion of Buddhist influence too far. It is customary in the West to draw rigid divisions between religions and denominations, but in India this has never really been the case. What seems likely is that numerous ideas were current in this period, which were made use of by those who followed the Buddha, and equally freely by Jains, Vedāntists and others. One might even argue that the Buddha borrowed his ideas from the Yoga teachings he encountered on his travels, but again this type of assertion is probably too simplistic.

1–2: KRIYĀ YOGA

1. *tapaḥ-svādhyāyeśvara-praṇidhānāni kriyā-yogaḥ,*
   Kriyā Yoga, yoga based on action, consists of religious austerity, recitation of the Vedas, and worship of the Lord.

2. *samādhi-bhāvanārthaḥ kleśa-tanū-karaṇārthaś ca,*
   The goal of Kriyā Yoga is to achieve the state of *samādhi*, and put an end to afflictions.

The opening two *sūtras* of the *Sādhana-pāda* introduce a new concept in the form of Kriyā Yoga, which is defined as consisting of acts of austerity, Vedic recitation, and worship of the Deity, *tapa, svādhyāya* and *īśvara*-praṇidh*āna*. The word *kriyā* comes from the verb *kṛ*, meaning to do or to act (which is also the root of the word karma), and *kriyā* usually means action or work. Kriy*ā* Yoga could be understood as an alternative form of Yoga, but it is probably better to understand the phrase as meaning action that is performed by Yoga practitioners. In other words, *tapa, svādhyāya* and *iśvara-praṇidhāna* may not be an intrinsic part of the limbs of Yoga, but they are also undertaken by *yogins*, and they will also help to induce the state of *samādhi* considered at the conclusion of the previous chapter. In fact the topic of Kriy*ā* Yoga is not pursued beyond these two verses, which provide the impetus for a new topic with the assertion that Kriy*ā* Yoga is performed to bring about the cessation of affliction. On the basis of that statement, Patañjali now turns to consider the afflictions in more detail.

3–9: THE AFFLICTIONS THAT KRIYA YOGA OVERCOMES

3. *avidyāsmitā-rāga-dveṣābhiniveśāḥ kleśāḥ,*
   The afflictions are ignorance, egotism, hankering, aversion, and attachment to life.

4. *avidyā kṣetraṃ uttareṣāṃ*
   prasupta-tanu-vicchinnodārāṇām,
   Ignorance is the basis of the other afflictions, whether they be dormant, slightly developed, occasional, or active.

5. *anityāśuci-duḥkhānātmasu nitya-śuci-sukhātma-khyātir avidyā,*
   Ignorance can be defined as regarding the temporary as permanent, the impure as pure, distress as pleasure, and thinking that which is not the self to be the self.

6. *dṛg-darśana-śaktyor ekātmatevāsmitā,*
   Egotism is in effect to misunderstand the seer to be the power of seeing.

7. *sukhānuśayī rāgaḥ,*
   Passion is the consequence that follows pleasure.

8. *duḥkhānuśayī dveṣaḥ,*
   Aversion is the consequence that follows suffering.

9. *sva-rasa-vāhī viduṣo 'pi tathārūḍho 'bhiniveśaḥ,*
   Even amongst men of wisdom, the longing for life flows of its own accord, and hence is firmly established.

Picking up on the mention of afflictions to be overcome, found in *sūtra* 2, the text now defines these in more detail. Firstly, they are listed as ignorance, egotism, hankering, aversion, and attachment to life. From reading this list, it is clearly apparent that they are not directly ways in which we suffer, but rather they are the causal factors that bring about the suffering we must endure.

Amongst these causal factors, it is *avidyā*, ignorance, which is the root cause upon which all the others are based. *Avidyā* is very specifically defined here as the failure to understand our true spiritual identity. Because of this ignorance, we see our identity in terms of the body and the mind, and seek pleasure through the gratification of body and mind. But these identities we currently hold are only temporary, confined to a single birth, and are not a reflection of the true self, which is eternal. They are impure and subject to contamination from the world, whilst the true self cannot be touched by the world in which it currently exists. And the pleasure sought through gratification of the body and mind is in fact simply a cause of distress, for all such pleasure is temporary, limited, and ultimately a source of frustration.

It is because of this ignorance of the *ātman* as the true self that the other *kleśas* appear. Firstly there is *asmitā*, the false sense of self, which relates to seeing oneself as body and mind rather than as the true seer, the *ātman* that is beyond the senses. Then there is *rāga*, the passion we have for renewed indulgence once a certain type of pleasure has been enjoyed; and the antithesis of *rāga* is *dveṣa*, the aversion or hatred we feel for anything (or anyone) which has caused us distress. And finally there is the longing for life, inherent in all beings, which, because death is inevitable, also becomes a cause of suffering.

This then is Patañjali's analysis of suffering, in which he follows other Indian thinkers by recognising ignorance of one's true identity as the ultimate causal factor. The *Yoga Sūtras* now makes it clear that these afflictions can be overcome, before offering a brief consideration of the manner in which the unfolding of karma is a factor in human suffering.

10–11: THE AFFLICTIONS CAN BE OVERCOME

10. *te pratiprasava-heyāḥ sūkṣmāḥ,*
    By turning them back to their original source, these afflictions can be overcome whilst still in their subtle form.

11. *dhyāna-heyās tad-vṛttayaḥ,*
    Even when they are active, they can be overcome through meditation.

It is a little difficult to establish exactly what is being presented here as the process by which the afflictions are overcome. *Sūtras* 1 and 2 gave a clear account of Kriyā Yoga as one method by which they can be restricted, but here we seem to have an alternative process defined as *pratiprasava*, the reversing or turning back of the afflictions whilst they are in a subtle form. It is hard to say exactly what this means though it might simply be an indication that if *avidyā* is addressed then the other afflictions based on *avidyā* will inevitably withdraw from their state of overt manifestation. What is clear is that the afflictions can be addressed whilst still in a subtle or non-overt form by means of *pratiprasava*, reversing the flow, or if they are already active by means of *dhyāna*, meditation. Beyond this, it is hard to be more definite in interpreting these *sūtras*.

12–14: THE AFFLICTIONS AS THE CAUSE OF KARMA

12. *kleśa-mūlaḥ karmāśayo dṛṣṭādṛṣṭa-janma-vedanīyaḥ,*
The accumulation of karma is based on these afflictions, and becomes manifest in seen and unseen births.

13. *sati mūle tad-vipāko jāty-āyur-bhogāḥ,*
As long as this basis exists, karma will come to fruition as the type of birth one takes, lifespan, and the fortune one experiences.

14. *te hlāda-paritāpa-phalāḥ puṇyāpuṇya-hetutvāt,*
These fruits then take the form of joy and misery, dependent on whether the karma is shaped by virtue or iniquity.

Here again we need to recall that these *kleśas*, or afflictions, are really causal factors that bring suffering upon us rather than the pains themselves. Now a further point is made, namely that the accumulation of karma is *kleśa-mūla*, in other words the *kleśas* are the root of karma. Now it is well known that the doctrine of karma indicates that the actions we perform will have a future result, dependent upon the nature of the action itself. So why would the *kleśas*, such as ignorance, egotism, passion etc., be described as the root of karma? The point must be that it is the *kleśas* that provide the impetus for action; because of *avidyā* we seek to gratify the body and mind in various ways, because of egotism we seek prestige and status through actions, and then passion for enjoyment causes us to act in a manner that will yield sensual delights. So in this sense the *kleśas* are not only the cause of our state of suffering, but also provide the impetus for action and then rebirth, as the karmic result arising from that action unfolds.

In *sūtra* 13, the ripening of karma is categorised in terms of the type of future birth we will attain, the lifespan within that bodily form, and also the good and bad fortune we will enjoy and endure; after all, even if one is born as a prince, events can still lead to a life of misery. And finally, in *sūtra* 14, we get a familiar reassertion of the essential doctrine of karma, to the effect that *puṇya karma*, righteous action, leads to *hlāda* or joy, whilst *a-puṇya karma*, unrighteous action, leads to *paritāpa* or suffering.

15–17: SUFFERING IS AN INHERENT FEATURE OF EXISTENCE

15. *pariṇāma-tāpa-saṁskāra-duḥkhair guṇa-vṛtti-virodhāc ca duḥkham eva sarvaṁ vivekinaḥ,*
Because of the misery caused by transformations, because of the suffering due to latent impressions, and because of the way in which one attribute of the world conflicts with another, the discriminating person sees all life as suffering.

16. *heyaṁ duḥkham anāgatam,*
It is, however, possible to prevent future suffering.

17. *draṣṭṛ-dṛśyayoḥ saṁyogo heya-hetuḥ,*
The means by which this is achieved is preventing contact between the seer and the world that is perceived.

Here we find what is in essence a reassertion of the first of the Buddha's four noble truths, that of *dukka* (*duḥkha*), which means that life in this world is inevitably beset by suffering. *Sūtra* 15 lists possible causes of this suffering, but concludes with the view of the *vivekins*, the wise ones, that *duḥkham eva sarvam*, everything is just misery. This is a rather depressing perspective on life, but it is one that is widely held in Indian religious thought, the point being that all the pleasures one achieves in life ultimately become sources of misery, as death and old age take it all away.

Swami Vivekananda once said, "Our philosophy begins with intense pessimism and ends with intense optimism," and this is reflected in this short passage. After the assertion *duḥkham eva sarvam*, it is stated that there is a remedy for this problem, which is described as *draṣṭṛ-dṛśyayoh saṁyogo heyaḥ*, the severing of the connection between the seer and the seen. Here of course the *draṣṭṛ*, the seer or the perceiver, is the *ātman*, and the *dṛśya*, the object of our perception, is the world. Hence the ending of the state of misery is achieved when the soul is freed from karma, and freed from the cycle of rebirth, or in Sāṁkhya terms when the *puruṣa*, the soul, is freed from its association with matter (*prakṛti*). Later in the *Yoga Sūtras* this state of liberation is referred to as *kaivalya*, literally aloneness or separation, but here it is presented as an introduction to the discussion of *sādhana*, the practice of Yoga, through which it can be attained.

18–27: LIBERATION FROM SUFFERING

18. *prakāśa-kriyā-sthiti-śīlaṃ bhūtendriyātmakaṃ bhogāpavargārthaṃ dṛśyam,*
    The world we perceive can have an identity that is illuminated, active, or still, and it consists of the material elements, and the senses of perception. It can be used either for enjoyment, or to achieve liberation from rebirth.

19. *viśeṣāviśeṣa-liṅga-mātrāliṅgāni guṇa-parvāṇi,*
The *guṇas*, the material attributes, can be designated as being specific and non-specific, as marked by clear characteristics, or as being free of such characteristics.

20. *draṣṭā dṛśi-mātraḥ śuddho 'pi pratyayānupaśyaḥ,*
Although the seer is entirely pure, and does nothing but observe, it still perceives the world in relation to this form of conceptualisation.

21. *tad-artha eva dṛśyasyātmā,*
The *ātman* is the only purpose behind the existence of the perceived world.

22. *kṛtārthaṃ prati naṣṭam apy anaṣṭaṃ tad-anya-sādhāraṇatvāt,*
Although the perceived world ceases to exist when the purpose of the *ātman* is achieved, it does not cease to exist entirely, for it continues to exist in relation to others.

23. *sva-svāmi-śaktyoḥ svarūpopalabdhi-hetuḥ saṃyogaḥ,*
The state of union between the seer and the perceived world exists in order to allow the seer to understand the true nature of the energies of the owner and the owned.

24. *tasya hetur avidyā,*
It is ignorance of this truth that is the cause of this state of union.

25. *tad-abhāvāt saṃyogābhāvo hānaṃ tad-dṛśeḥ kaivalyam,*
When that ignorance ceases the state of union also ceases. For the seer, this is the state known as *kaivalya*, separation from the world.

26. *viveka-khyātir aviplavā hānopāyaḥ,*
The continuous application of discriminative understanding is the means by which that cessation is achieved.

27. *tasya saptadhā prānta-bhūmiḥ prajñā,*
The realisation derived from that discriminative understanding is sevenfold, and reaches the ultimate point.

This passage builds on the reference to the *draṣṭṛ* and the *dṛśya*, the seer and the object that is seen, found in *sūtra* 17. It is quite clear that the *draṣṭṛ* is the *ātman* and the *dṛśya* is the material world it inhabits due to its embodiment, and which it perceives through the senses. Hence Patañjali is here reinforcing the essential distinction between *puruṣa* and *prakṛti*, spirit and matter, which lies at the heart of Sāṁkhya discourse.

Sūtras 18 and 19 consider the nature of the *dṛśya*, the material domain, although they do not make use of the usual Sāṁkhya enumerations of the elements of matter. The main point here is that the world can be used either for *bhoga*, the enjoyment of pleasure, or for *apavarga*, bringing about a cessation of worldly existence. *Sūtra* 19 refers to the *guṇas*, which, according to Sāṁkhya analysis, are the three fundamental qualities that pervade all aspects of matter. These are designated as *sattva*, or purity, *rajas*, or energy, and *tamas*, or darkness. Here, however, the reference is a little obscure, although the suggestion seems to be that the *guṇas* can have two contrasting forms, perhaps dependent on whether the world is seen as a source of pleasure, or as a means for achieving liberation from ignorance and rebirth. In his commentary, Vyasa draws upon some of the technical elements of Sāṁkhya philosophy in order to explain the *sūtra*, and, whilst his explanation is by no means implausible, it may well be an over-interpretation.

From *sūtra* 20, Patañjali turns his attention to the true self, the spiritual *draṣṭṛ*, the seer of the world. It is entirely pure, in the sense that it is untouched by the world, but still it perceives the world in terms of material transformations, because of its use of the senses. This *sūtra* is perhaps intended to explain how it is that the soul, which is entirely transcendent, still becomes prone to error and ignorance; the answer is that it perceives the world through the prism of the material senses.

Sūtras 21 to 23 then make an interesting point regarding the association of the *ātman* (the *draṣṭṛ*, the seer) with matter. It might be felt that matter is the enemy of the soul in the sense that it creates the bondage that binds the soul to ignorance and rebirth. However, this is not the case. Rather, matter is the means by which the soul can liberate itself from ignorance and rebirth, and in fact this is the only reason for its existence. This view is entirely consonant with the teachings of the *Sāṁkhya Kārikā*, and here we might note a few of the verses from that work:

58. Just as people perform acts to relieve their anxieties and longings, so matter in its non-manifest form is energised just for the purpose of *puruṣa mokṣa*, the liberation of the soul.
59. Just as a dancer will conclude her performance after displaying herself on stage, so Prakṛti (matter) displays herself to Puruṣa (the soul) and then withdraws.
60. The benevolent Prakṛti consists of three guṇas (qualities). She has no interest of her own to fulfil but becomes active to fulfil the object of the Puruṣa, who is beyond the guṇas.
61. In my view, there is nothing more delightful than Prakṛti. She recognises 'I have now been understood' and then withdraws from the vision of the Puruṣa.

(*Sāṁkhya Kārikā* of Ishvara Krishna)

In the *sūtras* here, we find Patañjali confirming this conclusion: matter exists for the sake of the soul's liberation, but it does not cease to exist when liberation occurs, for the obvious reason that there are still many unliberated souls existing under the influence of *avidyā*, ignorance, which *sūtra* 24 confirms as the actual cause of the soul's state of bondage. The material existence allows the soul to free itself from *avidyā*, and when it does so it achieves the state of *kaivalya*, absolute transcendence, where it is free from rebirth and suffering. The means by which ignorance is removed is here stated to be *viveka* (26), the knowledge that allows one to properly discriminate between what is the self and what is not the self; and the practice of Yoga is the means by which one becomes a *vivekin*, one who can discriminate correctly between the two. Here the realisation based on discriminative knowledge is said to be sevenfold, but no further explanation of this analysis is provided. Vyasa offers his own explanation of these seven stages, but there is no reason to presume that his interpretation is based on anything other than his own reasoning.

The important point we need to recognise from the first half of the *Samādhi-pāda* is that these *sūtras* locate the Yoga system at the heart of Indian religious discourse. The existence of the transcendent *ātman*, and the need to gain liberation from the world, are the fundamental notions on which Patañjali constructs his Yoga philosophy and Yoga teachings. The world is a place of suffering in which the effects of previous actions must be endured, but a solution can be found, and that solution is based on the notion of discriminative knowledge, which recognises the soul as being absolutely distinct from the world of matter. Here there is a close congruence with the teachings of Śaṅkarācārya, who similarly insists that knowledge alone is the key to *kaivalya*. Patañjali, however, holds to the Sāṁkhya view that the world is entirely real, and in fact exists not as the cause of the soul's bondage, but as the means by which its liberation can be achieved.

It is only after this philosophical understanding of the self and the world has been established that Patañjali feels able to begin his consideration of Yoga practice, perhaps because there is little point in outlining what needs to be done without clearly explaining the reason why this practice should be undertaken. Now that this has been established, the chapter proceeds on to its exposition of the eight limbs, the *aṣṭa aṅga*, of Yoga.

28–29: THE EIGHT LIMBS OF YOGA OUTLINED

28. *yogāṅgānuṣṭhānād aśuddhi-kṣaye jñāna-dīptir āviveka-khyāteḥ,*
When impurities dwindle due to one's practice of the limbs of Yoga, the light of true knowledge emerges, bringing with it discriminative understanding.

29. *yama-niyamāsana-prāṇāyāma-pratyāhāra-dhāraṇā-dhyāna-samādhayo'ṣṭāv aṅgāni,*
Restraints, observances, sitting postures, breath control, withdrawal of the senses, concentration of the mind, meditation, and complete absorption, are the eight limbs of Yoga.

Here then Patañjali reveals the central notion of his teachings on Yoga practice, the eight limbs that give rise to the name *aṣṭāṅga* that is frequently applied to this form of Yoga. As mentioned in *sūtra* 26, the *avidyā* that is the root cause of suffering can only be removed by *viveka*, discriminative knowledge. How then can this type of knowledge be acquired? The answer is given here; it is through *yoga-aṅga-anuṣṭhāna*, adherence to the limbs of Yoga. And these limbs are then listed as follows: *yama, niyama, āsana, prāṇāyāma, pratyāhāra, dhāranā, dhyāna,* and *samādhi*. Each of these eight will now be considered in turn with most attention being paid to the first two, *yama* and *niyama*.

30–32: THE YAMAS AND NIYAMAS LISTED

30. *ahiṃsā-satyāsteya-brahmacaryāparigrahā yamāḥ,*
The restraints are not harming, truthfulness, never stealing, celibacy, and not seeking ownership.

31. *jāti-deśa-kāla-samayānavacchinnāḥ sārvabhaumā mahā-vratam,*
These principles are not dependent on birth, place, time, or custom, but are equally applicable to all. Together they constitute the great vow.

32. *śauca-santoṣa-tapaḥ-svādhyāyeśvara-praṇidhānāni niyamāḥ,*
The observances are purity, contentment, austerity, recitation of the Veda, and worship of the Lord.

In these three *sūtras*, Patañjali provides a list of five *yamas* and then five *niyamas*. The usual translation for *yama* is a restraint, in the sense of avoiding an unwanted action, whilst *niyama* means an observance, in the sense of undertaking a beneficial type of action. The two lists are fairly straightforward, and more details are provided in the *sūtras* that follow, but at this stage we should note that the form of practice the *Yoga Sūtras* is advocating is tantamount to a serious spiritual vocation that involves an extreme level of commitment. Most people in the West and the East will find it virtually impossible to adhere even to these preliminary stages of Yoga, and may therefore feel that the whole process Patañjali is advocating is impractical for anyone other than the most ardent renunciant. In one sense this is true, but I think we should try to avoid the 'all or nothing' mentality that is somewhat alien to Indian thought, which tends towards the view that 'something is always better than nothing'. Perhaps it is more practical to regard the *yamas* and *niyamas* as ideals towards which the practitioner should strive rather than absolute prerequisites; after all, even Gandhi admitted that perfect *ahimsā* was impossible to achieve, and existed as an ideal, like Euclid's point.

The *yamas* are listed as *ahimsā*, not harming or non-violence, *satya*, speaking the truth or avoiding falsehood, *asteya*, not stealing, *brahmacharya*, celibacy, and *aparigraha*, having no sense of ownership. As these are forms of restraint, they primarily relate to actions that should be avoided, reflected in the fact that three of them are expressed in the negative (*a-himsā*, *a-steya* and *a-parigraha*). This kind of renounced lifestyle might be expected of priests or religious leaders, but Patañjali is adamant that persons of all backgrounds must adhere to this type of lifestyle if they are to successfully pursue the path of Yoga to its ultimate conclusion.

The *niyamas*, by contrast, are positive steps that the practitioner of Yoga should seek to adopt. These are listed as *śauca*, purity of both body and mind, *santoṣa*, contentment in the sense of not always seeking more than one already has, *tapas*, acts of religious austerity, *svādhyāya*, study and recitation of the Veda, and *īśvara*-praṇidh*āna*, devotion to *īśvara*, as was discussed earlier as an alternative means of stilling the movements of the mind.

Now that they have been listed, each of the *yamas* and each of the *niyamas* will be considered in turn.

33–34: ADVICE ON HOW TO OBSERVE YAMA AND NIYAMA

33. *vitarka-bādhane pratipakṣa-bhāvanam,*
When afflicted by ideas contrary to these observances, one should adopt an opposing mode of thought.

34. *vitarkā hiṃsādayaḥ kṛta-kāritānumoditā lobha-krodha-moha-pūrvakā mṛdu-madhyādhimātrā duḥkhājñānānanta-phalā iti pratipakṣa-bhāvanam,*

> Such an opposing mode of thought consists of regarding perverse tendencies such as harming others as producing unlimited misery and ignorance. This applies to all such tendencies, whether they are performed directly, performed through others, or simply approved of, whether they are based on greed, anger, or delusion, or whether they are adopted slightly, moderately, or with intensity.

As a preliminary, these two *sūtras* offer advice on how the practitioner should maintain resolve in adhering to *yama* and *niyama*. Essentially, the point being made here is that one should be mindful in the actions one performs, and in particular think carefully about the consequences of action. So if one feels drawn towards breaking the *yama* of *ahimsā*, then considering the suffering this will generate may act as a counter measure, and this same principle is to be applied to all the restraints and observances.

35–39: THE FIVE PRINCIPLES OF YAMA

35. *ahiṃsā-pratiṣṭhāyāṃ tat-saṃnidhau vaira-tyāgaḥ,*
When the principle of not harming is firmly established, any sense of enmity is given up by its presence.

36. *satya-pratiṣṭhāyāṃ kriyā-phalāśrayatvam,*
When the principle of truthfulness is firmly established, the results of action become certain.

37. *asteya-pratiṣṭhāyāṃ sarva-ratnopasthānam,*
When the principle of not stealing is firmly established, every type of gemstone approaches a person.

38. *brahmacarya-pratiṣṭhāyāṃ vīrya-lābhaḥ,*
When the principle of celibacy is firmly established, great potency is acquired.

39. *aparigraha-sthairye janma-kathantā-saṃbodhaḥ,*
When the principle of not seeking ownership becomes fixed, the details of previous births become known.

Each of these five sūtras deals with one of the *yamas* listed above in *sūtra* 30, and the main emphasis is on the positive result gained by adherence to each principle. A person who accepts the principle of *ahimsā* becomes free of enmity, perhaps in the sense that all antagonism towards others is removed from his own consciousness, or perhaps he is no longer regarded with enmity by any other creature. *Satya* makes the outcome of action certain; this may indicate that all endeavours meet with success, or it may simply mean that the outcome is certain because there is no dishonesty about the nature of the action, and the intention behind it.

Sūtras 37 to 38 seem to be looking ahead to the *Vibhūti-pāda*, the third chapter of the *Yoga Sūtras*, in which it is revealed that supernatural powers come to those who practise Yoga. Here we are told that a person who adheres strictly to the principle of *asteya*, not stealing, will be blessed with wealth of all kinds. Then if a person can adhere to a vow of celibacy, he will acquire *vīrya* or potency, an idea that is perhaps somewhat akin to Tantric teachings on sexual fluids and inner strength. Finally, if one adheres to the principle of *aparigraha*, having no sense of proprietorship, then he will come to understand the nature of previous births.

40–45: THE FIVE PRINCIPLES OF NIYAMA

40. *śaucāt svāṅga-jugupsā parair asaṃsargaḥ,*
As a result of practising purity, one develops distaste for one's own body, and avoids intimate bodily contact with others.

41. *sattva-śuddhi-saumanasyaikāgryendriya-jayātma-darśana-yogyatvāni ca,*

Through the principle of purity, one also acquires purification of one's existence, a genteel disposition, the ability to focus on a single object, mastery over the senses, and the ability to perceive the *ātman*.

42. *santoṣād anuttamaḥ sukha-lābhaḥ,*
As a result of contentment, the acquisition of happiness is unsurpassed.

43. *kāyendriya-siddhir aśuddhi-kṣayāt tapasaḥ,*
As a result of the dwindling of impurities due to acts of austerity, the body and senses acquire higher powers.

44. *svādhyāyād iṣṭa-devatā-samprayogaḥ,*
As a result of the recitation of the Veda, there is contact with the chosen deity.

45. *samādhi-siddhir īśvara-praṇidhānāt,*
As a result of worshipping the Lord, there is success in attaining the state of *samādhi*.

As with the *yamas*, the *niyamas* are now discussed in relation to the result they bring to one who is able to adhere to them. There are in fact six *sūtras* in the passage, as two are devoted to śau*cam*, purity, the first of the five. This is because the idea of *śaucam* relates to both bodily and mental purity, referred to respectively in *sūtras* 40 and 41. Bodily purity brings about an aversion to one's own body, and the bodies of others, and here we will be aware of the traditional Indian notion of ritual purity in which bodily fluids such as sweat, blood, or semen, are regarded as most impure. Mental purity, furthermore, brings about a benign disposition, and the ability to focus the mind on any object, including even the *ātman*, the true self. In this way the link between *niyama* and the goal of Yoga is very clearly established.

Santoṣa, or contentment, indicates a sense of satisfaction with whatever fortune brings, rather than constantly being in a state of agitation, and desire for material betterment. The point here is a very obvious one; if one can achieve this state of *santoṣa*, there will be a sense of complete happiness, for such a person is unrivalled in possessing everything he or she desires. *Tapas* is a term frequently encountered in Indian religious literature, often in relation to the extreme mortification of the body by means of which individuals seek extraordinary power, or the fulfilment of a particular desire. In the *Rāmāyaṇa*, for example, we read of how the demonic Rāvana undertook extreme *tapas* in order to gain the power to dominate the world, a situation that required a remedy in the form of the descent of Viṣṇu as the Rama *avatāra*. Here *tapas* seems to have a more benign meaning, although the idea is essentially the same; through acts of austerity the body and senses achieve a power far greater than is possible for ordinary people. Again we are in touch with the idea of the *yogin* acquiring supernatural abilities.

Svādhyāya is generally understood as the recitation of the Vedas, widely practised by brahminical communities in India, though it can also mean the quiet recitation of a single *mantra*. Here it is clearly the former meaning that is intended, as the recitation is said to bring one into contact with an *iṣṭa-devatā*, the deity of one's choice, which is almost certainly a reference to the Vedic gods glorified by the hymns of the *Saṁhitā* portion of the Veda. Finally, although it is given here as one of the *niyamas*, *īśvara*-praṇidhāna, devotion to God, is still presented in the same way as in the *Samādhi-pāda*, as an alternative means by which the perfection of Yoga can be achieved. This again reveals to us a fascinating insight into the link between Yoga and devotional Hinduism that was such a salient feature in the classical period, and can be observed most readily in the *Bhagavad-gītā*.

Now that the *yamas* and *niyamas* have been considered in relation to the rewards they bring, Patañjali moves forward with his discussion of the *Ashtāṅga Yoga*, and next considers the practice of *āsana*.

46–48: THE PRACTICE OF ĀSANA

46. *sthira-sukham āsanam,*
A sitting posture should be steady and comfortable.

47. *prayatna-śaithilyānanta-samāpattibhyām,*
This is achieved through the relaxation of exertion, and making contact with the unlimited.

48. *tato dvandvānabhighātaḥ,*
Then there is no further affliction from the dualities of existence.

The practice of *āsanas* is of course central to contemporary Yoga, and one might even say that it is primarily what modern Yoga is about. Patañjali, however, devotes only three *sūtras* to *āsana*, and there is no suggestion whatsoever that he is aware of, or is advocating, the variety of bodily postures undertaken as a part of Haṭha Yoga. Rather, *āsana* seems to be understood in terms of its literal meaning as simply the sitting posture one adopts in order to undertake the breathing and concentration exercises for the subsequent limbs. In describing the desired *ā*sana, sū*tra* 46 uses the words *sthira*, steady or firm, and *sukha,* meaning happy, or in this case comfortable, and the description here is very similar to that found in the *Bhagavad-gītā* (6.11), which also uses the word *sthiram.*

Sūtra 47 is slightly obscure in presenting the two features that allow for a steady and comfortable *āsana*. These are *prayatna-śaitilya* and *ananta-samāpatti. Prayatna-śaitilya* means a relaxation of effort, and probably suggests that the *āsana* adopted should be a natural one that does not require continuous effort to sustain. If one is to go on and practise the concentration of the mind, then having to make continuous exertion to hold a posture will clearly be problematic. We have already encountered the term *samāpatti* in the previous chapter (*sūtras* 41-46) where it was used to refer to the preliminary stage of *samādhi*. Hence *ananta-samāpatti* means absorption of the mind on the unlimited, which is presumably the *ātman*. It is not clear how this relates to the performance of *āsana*, but it may be that Patañjali is suggesting that when one achieves this high state of meditation, one's sitting posture naturally becomes steady and easy to hold. This would seem to be supported by *sūtra* 48, which indicates that when this is achieved dualities such as heat and cold, or happiness and distress, no longer affect the *yogin*, so that there is no difficulty in sustaining the desired *āsana*.

It is clear that whilst the *Yoga Sūtras* does include *āsana* as a part of the practice it advocates, it is not central to the process in the way that it becomes later in the Haṭha Yoga teachings. Patañjali's Yoga is not entirely distinct from contemporary practice, but it has undergone substantial modifications over the centuries and millennia.

49–53: THE PRACTICE OF PRĀṆAYĀMA

49. *tasmin sati śvāsa-praśvāsayor gati-vicchedaḥ prāṇāyāmaḥ,*
When this is achieved, the movement of the inhaled and exhaled breath can be restricted. This is *prāṇāyāma*.

50. *bāhyābhyantara-stambha-vṛttir deśa-kāla-saṁkhyābhiḥ paridṛṣṭo dīrgha-sūkṣmaḥ,*
The movement of the breath is external, internal, and then held steady. It can be observed in accordance with place, time, and number, and it can be either deep or shallow.

51. *bāhyābhyantara-viṣayākṣepī caturthaḥ,*
A fourth type of *prāṇāyāma* goes beyond the range of the external and internal movements.

52. *tataḥ kṣīyate prakāśāvaraṇam,*
In this way, the covering of illumination is diminished.

53. *dhāraṇāsu ca yogyatā manasaḥ,*
And the mind becomes ready for various forms of *dhāranā* (concentration).

In these five *sūtras*, Patañjali offers a brief insight into the fourth of the eight limbs, which is the practice of breath control, *prāṇāyāma*. We must first observe that very little by way of detail is provided, and it would be virtually impossible to engage in any form of *prāṇāyāma* exercise on the basis of this passage alone. Clearly it is not the author's intention to offer a detailed manual of regular practice.

So what do the *sūtras* tell us about *prāṇāyāma*? Firstly, it can be undertaken when the practice of *āsana* has been mastered, and then that it is about the inward breath, exhalation, and breath retention or suspension. These practices are undertaken in relation to the place and time, they are to be enumerated, and they can be done in a manner that is either deep or shallow. It is not entirely obvious what is meant here, but the indication is that a timed and enumerated rhythm should be imposed upon the breathing in terms of the inhalation of breath, its being held within the lungs, its expulsion, and then a pause before the next breath is inhaled. This can be done sometimes with very deep inhalations, and sometimes only lightly. Such breathing exercises will be familiar to most modern practitioners, and it seems clear that this imposition of regulation upon the breathing process is what Patañjali understands *prāṇāyāma* to consist of.

There is then a fourth element to the process, which goes beyond the internal and external breathing. It is not clear what this means, but it may be an indication that at a certain point the need for external control becomes unnecessary, and the *prāṇāyāma* becomes spontaneous and instinctive. Vyasa suggests that the fourth type of *prāṇāyāma* is where the movement of the breath is suspended entirely, but this is more than what the *sūtra* itself tells us.

Sūtras 52 and 53 then present the results that can be achieved through the successful practice of *prāṇāyāma*. Firstly, the *prakāśa āvaraṇa* is weakened. This presumably means the covering of ignorance that prevents the illumination of knowledge emerging, but it might possibly mean the spiritual light of the true self becoming increasingly apparent. And secondly, *prāṇāyāma* has a significant effect on the mind so that it becomes better able to perform the *dhāraṇā*, or concentration, discussed in the next chapter. The precise effect of *prāṇāyāma* upon the mind is not revealed, but it may be that it induces a state of profound tranquillity in which concentrated and precise focus becomes easier to achieve. The important point to note here is that for Patañjali, *prāṇāyāma* has a place in a sequence of practices that act as a preparation for the higher realisations of Yoga. It is not shown to have any other purpose beyond this.

54–55: THE PRACTICE OF PRATYĀHĀRA

54. *sva-viṣayāsamprayoge cittasya svarūpānukāra ivendriyāṇāṁ pratyāhāraḥ,*
    Pratyāhāra is where the senses end their contact with their respective objects, and assume the same nature as the mind.

55. *tataḥ paramā vaśyatendriyāṇām,*
    It is in this way that one gains absolute control over the senses.

The final two *sūtras* of Chapter 2 deal very briefly with the fifth of the *aṣṭāṅga*, namely *pratyāhāra*, which is usually understood to mean the withdrawal of the senses from external perception. This brevity is perhaps surprising as it is made quite clear in both the *Mahābhārata* and in the *Yoga*

Sūtras itself that the internal realisation of the true self, which is the goal of Yoga, is only possible when external, sensory perception is suspended.

Here the two *sūtras* do little more than provide a definition of what is meant by *pratyāhāra*, without offering any advice as to how it is to be achieved, nor giving any indication of the immediate results to be gained thereby. All that is said is that *pratyāhāra* is where the senses no longer make contact with the objects of perception (sound, form, aroma, flavour, and touch), and are withdrawn back into the mind. This withdrawal is the means by which the senses are brought under control.

Now five limbs of the eight have been delineated and briefly explained. The next chapter deals primarily with the results that can be derived through rigorously following this process, but before this topic can be considered it will be necessary to complete the present discussion by considering the final three limbs, *dhāraṇā*, *dhyāna* and *samādhi.*

CHAPTER 3: THE VIBHŪTI-PĀDA

THE word *vibhūti* usually means glories or opulence, and in this third chapter of the *Yoga Sūtras* Patañjali expounds at some length on the wonderful supernatural powers the adept can achieve through the practice of Yoga. So here *vibhūti* refers to the miraculous results that are gained through dedication to the practice previously outlined.

First, though, the discussion of the eight limbs of Yoga has to be concluded, and so the chapter begins with a brief explanation of what is meant by *dhāraṇā*, *dhyāna* and *samādhi*. These three final limbs are clearly closely related to one another, and throughout the main part of the chapter are considered almost as a single process, referred to as *saṁyama*. It is declared that *saṁyama* is the very essence of Yoga, standing above and beyond the first five limbs, for it is at this point that *citta-vṛtti-nirodha* is finally achieved.

From *sūtra* 14 onwards, the text takes a rather unexpected turn, as Patañjali begins to focus on the supernatural or magical powers the *yogin* acquires by applying the power of *saṁyama* to different objects of contemplation. A long list of such powers is given along with the means of acquiring each of them, but a careful reading of the chapter reveals that a fundamental distinction is to be drawn between powers that can be applied to this world, and those that help to achieve the goal of absolute transcendence, *kaivalya,* which takes the *yogin* entirely beyond the manifest world into the domain of the spirit. The movement of the text between these two outcomes is often rather subtle, and there are times when it is not entirely clear which of the two is being referred to, but on a number of occasions it is made wholly apparent that the magical powers acquired are not the highest goal of Yoga, and are in fact an obstacle in themselves to the attainment of *kaivalya*, which can only be achieved if and when such powers are renounced. This is one point we will look out for as we progress through the chapter.

Patañjali's discussion of magic and supernatural powers inevitably raises doubts in the rational mind about the authenticity of his teachings. People today are instinctively dubious about claims of miracles, and indeed one of the attractions of Yoga is that it is a form of spirituality that does not depend on faith in the supernatural, but rather on verifiable experience. So what then are we to make of the content of the *Vibhūti-Pāda*?

The treatises on Yoga in the *Bhagavad-gītā* and the *Mahābhārata* make no mention of these *vibhūtis*, although various narratives contained within the *Mahābhārata* refer to *yogins* possessing such powers. Moreover, in modern India the idea of saints and holy men being capable of supernatural feats is widely accepted, and at times even expected. Still, however, the question remains as to whether the claims made in this third chapter somehow undermine the validity of the *Yoga Sūtras* as a whole. After all, if Patañjali is deemed to be making impossible claims for Yoga here, why should we think that he is doing anything different in the other sections of his work?

There is no obvious solution to this question and different individuals will reach different conclusions. Some may feel that to exclude the possibility of supernatural occurrences is overly dogmatic, while others may hold the view that even if the claims made here are exaggerations based on cultural perspectives, this does not invalidate other teachings on Yoga that can be substantially verified on the basis of personal experience. I do not have any clear cut solutions to offer on this point, but I do think the question is one that we need to raise and consider in developing a full understanding of the teachings offered by the *Yoga Sūtras*.

1–3: DHĀRAṆĀ, DHYĀNA, AND SAMĀDHI

1. *deśa-bandhaś cittasya dhāraṇā,*
   Dhāraṇā is the fixing of the mind on a particular point.

2. *tatra pratyayaika-tānatā dhyānam,*
   Dhyāna is where the focus of the mind remains constantly on that single object.

3. *tad evārtha mātra-nirbhāsaṃ svarūpa-śūnyam iva samādhiḥ,*
   Samādhi is where the object alone illuminates the consciousness, and appears devoid of any external form.

These three opening *sūtras* appear to conclude Patañjali's discourse on the *aṣṭāṅga*, the eight limbs of Yoga, though of course they are grouped together and discussed further in the following *sūtras*, under the joint heading of *saṁyama*. And even here, it is readily apparent that *dhāraṇā, dhyāna* and *samādhi* are very closely connected. *Dhāraṇā* is defined succinctly as the *deśa-bandha* of the *citta*, the binding of the *citta* to a single place, in other words concentration on one point alone. When that *dhāraṇā* becomes constant and unwavering, it is then identified as *dhyāna*; one might therefore say that *dhyāna* is the successful and unwavering execution of *dhāraṇā*.

Then when the process is carried a step further, the concentration becomes so intense that the object alone fills one's consciousness in a manner that goes beyond thought processes related to the attributes of that object. This total absorption of the mental faculties, beyond the stage of conscious thought, is what is referred to as *samādhi*. If we refer back to Patañjali's original definition of Yoga, we can see that *samādhi* is certainly equivalent to the *citta-vṛtti-nirodha*, the stilling of the movements of the mind, he originally referred to. It is perhaps noteworthy, however, that *samādhi* is here described as a state of mind, and a state of consciousness; it is not necessarily applied to the spiritual realisation that dispels *avidyā*, ignorance, and thereby grants *kaivalya*. *Samādhi* can be employed as a means of achieving *kaivalya*, but *kaivalya* is not an inevitable concomitant of *samādhi*, as will be made clear by the discussion of *vibhūti* later in this chapter.

4–8: SAṀYAMA, THE ESSENCE OF YOGA PRACTICE

4. *trayam ekatra saṁyamaḥ,*
   When these three are applied to a single object, this is known as *saṁyama*.

5. *taj-jayāt prajñālokaḥ,*
   When mastery in *saṁyama* is achieved, one's understanding is illuminated.

6. *tasya bhūmiṣu viniyogaḥ,*
   This process is mastered by progressive stages.

7. *trayam antar-aṅgaṃ pūrvebhyaḥ,*
   These three are the very essence of Yoga, transcending the previous limbs.

8. *tad api bahir-aṅgaṃ nirbījasya,*
   Though they in turn are external to the Yoga that is without seed.

These five *sūtras* then assert that the final three limbs of the *aṣṭāṅga* are known collectively as *saṁyama*, and from this point onwards are taken virtually as a single process. *Sūtra* 5 gives us the primary result gained through *saṁyama*, namely *prajñā aloka*, the illumination of wisdom or understanding. As the cause of the bondage of the soul has already been designated as *avidyā*, ignorance, we can see how *saṁyama* is to be understood as the means by which the soul gains release from bondage into the state of *kaivalya*.

Sūtra 6 informs the reader that this highest achievement of Yoga will be achieved gradually and by stages; in other words one should not expect immediate success. It is in fact the essence of, and purpose behind, the previous five stages of practice, which again tells us something about the way in which Patañjali perceives the significance of *ā*sana, *prāṇāyāma* and *pratyāhara*. But finally we are told that there is a level of attainment beyond even the *samādhi* achieved through perfect *dhārāṇa* and *dhyāna*. It seems that because there is an object on which the mind is focused in *dhārāṇa* and *dhyāna*, the *samādhi* they ultimately produce is *sa-bīja samādhi*. This, however, is just the external form of the ultimate level of realisation, referred to as *nir-bīja*, which is that of pure, changeless consciousness, in which there is no object or 'seed' of any kind.

9–13: THE TRANSFORMATIONS BROUGHT ABOUT BY SAṀYAMA

9. *vyutthāna-nirodha-saṁskārayor abhibhava-prādurbhāvau nirodha-kṣaṇa-cittānvayo nirodha-pariṇāmaḥ,*

   The change brought about by restricting the movements of the mind consists of the overpowering of the latent impressions as they arise, and the appearance of the latent impressions of restraint. This condition of the mind arises at the moment when its movement is restricted.

10. *tasya praśānta-vāhitā saṁskārāt,*
A flow of tranquillity arises from this new form of latent impression.

11. *sarvārthataikāgratayoḥ kṣayodayau cittasya samādhi-pariṇāmaḥ,*
When the focus of the mind on all the objects of the world declines, and the state of single-mindedness arises, this is the transformation of consciousness towards *samādhi.*

12. *tataḥ punaḥ śāntoditau tulya-pratyayau cittasyaikāgratā-pariṇāmaḥ,*
The transformation of the mind towards one-pointedness occurs when an idea takes the same form whether at peace or arising.

13. *etena bhūtendriyeṣu dharma-lakṣaṇāvasthā pariṇāmā vyākhyātāḥ,*
In this way, I have now explained the transformations of the fundamental nature, the characteristic marks, and the condition of the material elements and the senses.

The central theme of the third chapter of the *Yoga Sūtras* is the results acquired through mastery of *saṁyama*, the final three limbs of the eight limbs of Yoga, which in turn is only possible through mastery of the previous five. Before Patañjali gets fully into this discourse, however, he begins by giving some explanation of how it is that *saṁyama* can achieve the remarkable results he is about to describe. Hence in these five *sūtras* he attempts to explain something of what happens to the human consciousness when *saṁyama* is finally perfected.

The key theme here is *pariṇāma*, the transformation of the consciousness that *saṁyama* brings about, so that the mind of the *yogin* is of a different order to the minds of others. The essence of this transformation is outlined in *sūtra* 9 in relation to the *saṁskāras*, the latent impressions left upon the mind as a result of the experiences we undergo and the actions we perform. Through *saṁyama* these *saṁskāras* are subtly eroded, and replaced by new *saṁskāras*, the *saṁskāras* of restraint, which have the effect of unleashing a flood of tranquillity, if that is not too much of an oxymoron. Naturally, therefore, we presume that these new *saṁskāras* are desirable, but let us not forget the indication of *sūtra* 8, which refers to a *nir-bīja* state beyond that referred to here. It seems likely that although the *saṁskāras* of restraint are certainly desirable, they are still *saṁskāras* that must also be transcended if one is to reach the *nir-bīja* level of consciousness.

The transformation is further elaborated upon in *sūtras* 11 and 12: it is based on ending the perception of objects in the external world, and this form of perception being replaced by a state of mind where the focus is on one object alone. Perception is no longer external but is turned exclusively inwards, whilst the processes of thought and conceptualisation are brought to an end. The object of thought enters the conscious mind but it never leaves the dormant state of conception. And again we can regard these *sūtras* as an elaboration on what exactly is meant by the phrase *citta-vṛtti-nirodha*, and the way in which it changes the consciousness of an individual.

14–16: KNOWLEDGE OF PAST AND FUTURE ACHIEVED THROUGH SAṀYAMA

14. *śāntoditāvyapadeśya-dharmānupātī dharmī,*
Something can be said to possess a fundamental nature when that nature is present whether the object is at peace, arising, or devoid of any discernible mark.

15. *kramānyatvaṃ pariṇāmānyatve hetuḥ,*
It is differences in the nature of progression that cause differences in the nature of the transformation achieved.

16. *pariṇāma-traya-saṁyamād atītānāgata-jñānam,*
Through *saṁyama* on the three transformations, one acquires knowledge of the past and future.

Although these *sūtras* are clearly describing how a type of *saṁyama* brings the miraculous ability to know the past and future, the full meaning of the text is obscure, although Vyasa is helpful here in providing a viable explanation. He suggests that the words *śānta*, at peace, *udita*, arising, and *avyapadeśya*, without discernible mark, mentioned in 14, actually mean past, present and future, and that it is this temporal change that gives rise to the transformation of an object. If this view is accepted, then it becomes more apparent as to why *saṁyama* on that process of transformation should produce the mystic ability to discern past and future.

The indication of this and subsequent passages is that once the ability to achieve the state of *saṁyama* has been mastered, it can be applied at will to a range of different objects. And all that Patañjali is doing in this chapter is indicating the type of *saṁyama* that is to be applied in order to achieve supernatural powers of various types. This is the first in a lengthy list of such powers, the power of clairvoyance frequently claimed by fortune-tellers and soothsayers. Going through the chapter, one is struck by the wonderful array of the mystic attributes *yogins* are said to acquire, and as such abilities are so rarely encountered either in India or the West, one must presume that the power of *saṁyama* is attained very infrequently by *yogins.*

17–22: FIVE FURTHER POWERS DESCRIBED

17. *śabdārtha-pratyayānām itaretarādhyāsāt saṅkaras tat pravibhāga-saṁyamāt sarva-bhūta-ruta-jñānam,*
Because of the superimposition of one onto the other, the word, its meaning, and the concept it represents become confused, but by the application of *saṁyama* to the distinctions between these, one acquires knowledge of the speech of all beings.

18. *saṁskāra-sākṣāt-karaṇāt pūrva-jāti-jñānam,*
Through the direct perception of latent impressions on the mind, one gains knowledge of one's previous births.

19. *pratyayasya para-citta-jñānam,*
And through the direct perception of the overt concept, one acquires knowledge of other people's minds.

20. *na ca tat sālambanaṃ tasyāviṣayī bhūtatvāt,*
But this knowledge does not apply to the nature of the object the other is thinking of, as this is not the object of the practitioner's perception.

21. *kāya-rūpa-saṁyamāt tad-grāhya-śakti-stambhe cakṣuḥ-prakāśāsaṁprayoge 'ntardhānam,*
Through *saṁyama* on the form of the body when its ability to be perceived is suspended and there is no contact with the illumination of eyesight, one acquires the power to become invisible.

22. *sopakramaṁ nirupakramaṁ ca karma tat-saṁyamād aparānta-jñānam ariṣṭebhyo vā,*

Karma may or may not have yet produced a result. By *saṁyama* on both types of karma, one acquires knowledge of the time of death. Such knowledge can also be derived from omens.

From this point onwards, the *Vibhūti-Pāda* gets into its central line of discourse, explaining *sūtra* by *sūtra* how *saṁyama* on a different object will produce a certain supernatural power. In truth, the chapter now reads rather like a list, and as a result I do not feel we need to discuss its content in the same depth as elsewhere. What I particularly want to highlight, however, is where Patañjali moves from revealing the worldly (albeit supernatural) powers acquired through *saṁyama* to considering the higher, spiritual attainments that lead ultimately to *kaivalya*, release from rebirth.

Here five powers are given in six *sūtras*, as *sūtra* 20 provides some further information on the power to read minds, presented in 19. The five mystical abilities are knowledge of the speech of different creatures, gaining knowledge of one's previous births, being able to read other people's minds, the power to become invisible, and being able to determine the time of one's death. In each case, it is *saṁyama* on a particular object that grants these powers, though in several instances the precise nature of the object of the required *saṁyama* is obscure. Let us now proceed through the full list of the higher powers that Patañjali claims can be achieved through Yoga practice.

23–27: FIVE FURTHER POWERS

23. *maitryādiṣu balāni,*
    By *saṁyama* on good will and other such qualities, one acquires related powers.

24. *baleṣu hasti-balādīni,*
    By *saṁyama* on the power of an elephant and other animals, one acquires their strength.

25. *pravṛtty-āloka-nyāsāt sūkṣma-vyavahita-viprakṛṣṭa-jñānam,*
By utilising the illumination of one's practice, one acquires knowledge of things that are subtle, concealed, and far distant.

26. *bhuvana-jñānaṃ sūrye saṁyamāt,*
Knowledge of different worlds is acquired through *saṁyama* on the sun.

27. *candre tārā-vyūha-jñānam,*
Saṁyama on the moon brings knowledge of the position of the stars.

Here the five powers Patañjali describes are *balāni,* simply powers or abilities, coming to possess the strength of an elephant, or some other powerful beast, being able to acquire knowledge of hidden or distant matters, coming to possess knowledge of other worlds, and then acquiring knowledge of the movements of the stars. Again the application of *saṁyama* to a designated object is given as the means, although some difference might be detected in *sūtra* 25 where *nyāsa,* here meaning fixing upon, is presented as the means.

28–32: FIVE FURTHER POWERS

28. *dhruve tad-gati-jñānam,*
Saṁyama on the polestar, Dhruva, brings knowledge of the movement of the stars.

29. *nābhi-cakre kāya-vyūha-jñānam,*
Saṁyama on the navel brings knowledge of the workings of the body.

30. *kaṇṭha-kūpe kṣut-pipāsā-nivṛttiḥ,*
Through *saṁyama* on the pit of the throat, hunger

and thirst cease to have any effect.

31. *kūrma-nāḍyāṃ sthairyam,*
Through *saṁyama* on the tortoise channel, one acquires steadiness.

32. *mūrdha-jyotiṣi siddha-darśanam,*
Through *saṁyama* on the light within the head, one becomes able to see higher beings.

Continuing with the established pattern of the discourse, Patañjali here firstly reveals that *saṁyama* on Dhruva, or the polestar, brings the adept knowledge of the movements of the stars, something that would be useful for astrological purposes. Then by applying the same intense mental absorption to one's navel, or *nābhi*, he acquires a detailed understanding of the functioning of the organs of the body. *Saṁyama* on the pit of the throat removes the influence of hunger and thirst, and *sthairya*, or steadiness, is acquired by the *yogin* who applies his *saṁyama* to the *kūrma-nāḍi*, an interesting and rather obscure reference.

Tantric and Hatha Yoga employ ideas of a subtle anatomy based on *cakras* or energy centres, and a network of channels along which subtle energy is passed. Patañjali's teachings on Yoga are almost entirely preoccupied with mental processes, and he displays no interest whatsoever in these Tantric notions, so it is interesting to observe here that he was aware, at least to some degree, of the concept of the *nāḍi* as a channel within the body, although it is not clear whether this is a vein, a nerve, or one of the subtle channels. The word *kūrma* means a tortoise or turtle, and so the *kūrma-nāḍi* is the tortoise channel, but we are given no further insight as to exactly what this means.

Sūtra 32 refers to the power to perceive higher beings. The traditional Indian understanding is that the world is populated by gods and spirits of many different types. Some of these exist in higher worlds, but others are present amongst us in invisible forms, and may at times have a positive or malefic influence upon our lives. Here it is stated that when the practice of *saṁyama* is applied to the *mūrdha-jyotis*, the light or illumination within the head, it becomes possible to perceive these higher beings. Again it is rather difficult to say exactly what is meant by *mūrdha-jyotis*, and Vyasa offers very little by way of guidance.

33–37: THE REJECTION OF HIGHER POWERS

33. *prātibhād vā sarvam,*
Otherwise, all things can be acquired through the awakening of intuitive knowledge.

34. *hṛdaye citta-saṁvit,*
Through *saṁyama* on the heart, one acquires understanding of the thought processes.

35. *sattva-puruṣayor atyantāsaṅkīrṇayoḥ pratyayāviśeṣo bhogaḥ parārthatvāt svārtha-saṁyamāt puruṣa-jñānam,*
Worldly pleasure is based on the misidentification of *sattva* with *puruṣa*, which are entirely distinct. Through *saṁyama* on the true identity, one acquires knowledge of the *puruṣa*.

36. *tataḥ prātibha-śrāvaṇa-vedanādarśāsvāda-vārtā jāyante,*
When this state is achieved, intuitive knowledge and higher powers of hearing, touch, seeing, tasting, and smelling arise.

37. *te samādhāv upasargā vyutthāne siddhayaḥ,*
When these higher powers arise, however, they are an obstacle to *samādhi*.

It may not be immediately obvious, but I think that what we have here marks a change in the line of discussion, and that Patañjali is now speaking about the higher spiritual goal that can be achieved when *saṁyama* is properly applied. Hence we may need to consider the meaning of these *sūtras* in a little more detail.

Sūtra 33 is rather terse and can be easily passed over in the flow of the chapter, but what it says is that all powers can be achieved through *prātibha*, a word which means intuitive rather than reasoned knowledge. This may refer to a higher realisation that brings with it all the powers referred to in this chapter, as indicated in *sūtra* 36, but we cannot be certain on that point. Similarly, the *citta-saṁvit*, meaning understanding of the *citta*, mentioned in 34, as the result of applying *saṁyama* to the heart, may just be another of the powers, but it could possibly indicate something more in terms of a higher form of realisation.

When we move on to *sūtra* 35, however, we can be more definite in concluding that Patañjali has now progressed to a different idea. Here he states that *bhoga*, enjoyment of the world, is based on the false identification of *sattva* and *puruṣa*, and in this case I think it is safe to presume that *sattva* refers to the material body and mind, a sense in which the term is often used in Sāṁkhya discourse. Pleasure is gained through the gratification of the body and mind, but only as long as one mistakenly regards oneself in terms of this identity, and remains unaware of *puruṣa*, one's true spiritual identity. And here the point would be that the material powers previously listed all fall within the domain of *bhoga*, and hence form a part of the illusion, the *avidyā*, that forms the main barrier to *kaivalya*.

The illusion is dispelled by *puruṣa-jñāna*, knowledge of the *puruṣa*, which can be acquired when *saṁyama* is employed for this higher purpose. The indication of *sūtra* 36 is that when this realisation of the *puruṣa* is attained through the appropriate *saṁyama*, then all the higher powers of the senses previously referred to are achieved as well. However, these worldly abilities must not be allowed to cause a distraction, and are to be recognised as obstacles in the quest to achieve full *samādhi*. This statement of *sūtra* 37 might seem to be a little odd, as *samādhi* is one of the three components of *saṁyama*, and the powers that have been listed are achieved by means of *saṁyama*.

There are, I think, two points to note here. Firstly, Patañjali seems quite clear in stressing that the supernatural abilities he has described are not the highest goal of Yoga practice, and are in fact to be regarded as obstacles to the attainment of that highest goal, which is *kaivalya*. And secondly, one might suggest that the state of *samādhi* referred to in 37 is probably the *nirbīja samādhi* mentioned earlier in *sūtra* 8, of which the eight limbs are just an external form. The mystical powers are achieved through *sa-bīja samādhi*, but the higher spiritual goal of *kaivalya* is reached through *nirbīja samādhi*.

38–42: FIVE FURTHER POWERS

38. *bandha-kāraṇa-śaithilyāt pracāra-saṁvedanāc ca cittasya para-śarīrāveśaḥ,*
By loosening the causes of bondage, and by perceiving the movements of the mind, one can enter within another person's body.

39. *udāna-jayāj jala-paṅka-kaṇṭakādiṣv asaṅga utkrāntiś ca,*
By controlling the *udāna* air, one can raise oneself upwards and remain untouched by water, mud, thorns, and other obstacles.

40. *samāna-jayāj jvalanam,*
By controlling the *samāna* air, one's body becomes illuminated.

41. *śrotrākāśayoḥ sambandha-saṁyamād divyaṁ śrotram,*
Through *saṁyama* on the connection between hearing and space, one acquires celestial powers of hearing.

42. *kāyākāśayoḥ sambandha-saṁyamāl laghu-tūla-samāpatteś cākāśa-gamanam,*
Through *saṁyama* on the connection between the body and space, and absorbing oneself in the lightness of cotton, one gains the power to travel through the sky.

Here, however, we are clearly returning to the previous theme of the supernatural powers that can be acquired through Yoga practice, and this moving back and forth can be a little confusing. It might even appear that Patañjali does not want to draw a clear distinction between these magical abilities, and the spiritual goals that lead ultimately to liberation from misery and rebirth.

Given this rather curious juxtaposition of ideas, can we then be certain as to whether Patañjali is saying that the powers are an obstacle to spiritual progress? Certainly *sūtra* 37 appears to be making this point, but this could be taken as referring only to the higher sensory faculties mentioned in *sūtra* 36, as it has been made clear throughout that the senses must be withdrawn for *samādhi* to be achieved. Then if we look ahead we will see that *sūtra* 50 also advocates the renunciation (*vairāgya*) of supernatural abilities, but again we cannot be sure that this does not apply solely to those mentioned in *sūtra* 49.

It is hard to be certain on this point, and there is undoubtedly a degree of ambivalence in both the structure of the discourse, and in terms of the precise meaning of the relevant *sūtras*. It is, I think, legitimate to say that the *Yoga Sūtras* states that the supernatural powers must be renounced lest they become a distraction from the true goal, but we should be at least a little cautious in pressing this view too far; and it is noteworthy that Vyasa does not appear to share this perspective.

Here we might also note that Yogic techniques apart from *saṁyama*, notably different forms of *prāṇāyāma*, are presented as a means through which different powers can be acquired. Firstly though, reference is made to the ability to enter another person's body, a magical feat quite commonly encountered in Indian literature, including the biography of Śaṅkarācārya. *Sūtras* 39 and 40 describe the powers of levitation and illumination, which are acquired through mastery of the *udāna* and *samāna* airs respectively. *Sūtra* 41 states that *divya śrotra*, celestial hearing, is acquired when *saṁyama* is applied to the connection between space and hearing. And then 42 states that *saṁyama* on the connection between space and the body, along with *samāpatti* on the lightness of cotton, will enable the *yogin* to fly through the sky. Again this mystical ability is one that is frequently referred to in the numerous Indian narratives in which great *yogins* appear, and it is interesting to note that the Transcendental Meditation group uses this *sūtra* as a part of its 'Yogic Flying Sidhi' programme.

43–46: ACHIEVING THE PERFECT BODILY FORM

43. *bahir-akalpitā-vṛttir mahā-videhā tataḥ prakāśāvaraṇa-kṣayaḥ,*
The great detachment from the body, the *mahā-videha*, occurs when the movements of the mind are no longer directed outwards. When this is achieved, the covering of illumination dwindles.

44. *sthūla-svarūpa-sūkṣmānvayārthavattva-saṁyamād bhūta-jayaḥ,*
Through *saṁyama* on their gross form, their essential nature, the subtle form, their relationships

and functions, one acquires mastery over the material elements.

45. *tato 'ṇimādi-prādurbhāvaḥ kāya-sampat-tad-dharmānabhighātaś ca,*
At this point, powers such as making the body minute also appear; the body achieves a perfect state, and the limitations imposed by its inherent nature are overcome.

46. *rūpa-lāvaṇya-bala-vajra-saṁhananatvāni kāya-sampat,*
The perfect state of the body includes beauty, grace, strength, and the hardness of diamond.

As we approach the conclusion of the chapter, we now reach the point where the highest type of supernatural powers are described in terms of the *kāya-saṁvit*, the perfect bodily form. At this stage, the *yogin* is transformed from man to superman, something inconceivable to the Western mind but a common feature of Indian literature, and still widely believed in by the people of India.

Firstly, the external movements of the mind, the external *vṛttis*, are restrained, leading to what is referred to as the *mahā-videha*. This term literally means the great detachment from the body, and according to Vyasa it indicates that when one enters the deepest state of meditation all awareness of the body ceases, for one's perception is entirely internal. At this point the coverings of illusion begin to disappear. Then when *saṁyama* is applied to the different features of the great elements, defined in Sāṁkhya thought as earth, water, air, fire, and space, mastery over these elements is gained. It is not exactly clear what this means, but as the body is said to consist of these elements, there is an obvious link to the development of the *kāya-saṁvit*, the perfect body referred to in *sūtras* 45 and 46.

It is *bhūta-jaya*, mastery over the material elements, that leads to the attainment of powers such as *animā*, the ability to become minutely small, and then the *kāya-saṁvit*, the perfect body. Although Patañjali does not have much to say about *animā* and the associated *siddhis*, they are widely referred to elsewhere in Indian religious literature as the main powers achieved through Yoga. Here we just have the phrase *animādi*, meaning *animā* and the others, suggesting that Patañjali presumes a knowledge of what the other *siddhis* are.

The usual listing of the eight *siddhis* is as follows:

1. *animā*, the ability to become minutely small
2. *mahimā*, the ability to become large in size
3. *laghimā*, the ability to become light and float through the air
4. *garimā*, the ability to become heavy and immovable
5. *prāpti*, the ability to acquire objects from distant places
6. *prākāmya*, the ability to do whatever one desires without restriction
7. *vaśitva*, the ability to bring other beings under one's control
8. *īśitva*, the ability to achieve mastery over the world

Clearly some of these *siddhis* have already been referred to as the results achieved through different types of *saṁyama*. The reference here is interesting, however, as the *siddhis* are more usually referred to in texts relating to Tantric Yoga, and the fact that Patañjali displays and presumes a familiarity with them gives a slight hint that he may have had a greater knowledge of Tantra than he chooses to reveal in the *Yoga Sūtras*.

Related to the acquisition of the *animādi siddhis* is the notion of the *kāya-saṁvit*. The body is transformed so that the *yogin* experiences none of the restraints or limitations that affect the lives of other people. His form is now elegant and beautiful, yet filled with power, and as hard and impenetrable as diamond. This state of existence seems to be the epitome of the physical achievement the *yogin* attains, transforming him into a godlike being, far beyond the conventional limitations imposed by the human condition.

47–49: THE ALTERNATIVE PATH OF SPIRITUAL AWAKENING

47. *grahaṇa-svarūpāsmitānvayārthavattva-saṁyamād indriya-jayaḥ,*
    Through *saṁyama* on their perception of objects, their inherent nature, the sense of ego, their relationship with other faculties, and their purpose, one achieves mastery over the senses.

48. *tato mano-javitvaṃ vikaraṇa-bhāvaḥ pradhāna-jayaś ca,*
    When the senses are mastered, the mind can act quickly, one's existence needs no external support, and one gains domination over matter.

49. *sattva-puruṣānyatā-khyāti-mātrasya sarva-bhāvādhiṣṭhātṛtvaṁ sarva-jñātṛtvaṁ ca,*
    When there is a full understanding of the distinction between matter and *puruṣa*, one acquires mastery over all that exists, and knowledge of all things as well.

I think that in these *sūtras* we can genuinely detect the beginning of a move from discussion of supernatural powers towards an emphasis on spiritual realisation, which the first two chapters proclaimed to be the true goal of Yoga. In a sense, the discussion of magical abilities reached its full conclusion in the references to *animā* and the other *siddhis*, and then the transformation of the body into the *kāya-saṁvit*. Here we should pay particular attention to the phrase *sattva-puruṣanyatā-khyāti*, which means revelation of the absolute distinction between *sattva* and *puruṣa*, matter and spirit, and be aware that in Sāṁkhya teachings this is the ultimate goal to be achieved, the goal that brings release from rebirth.

Firstly though, *sūtra* 47 states that *saṁyama* on the working of the senses brings *indriya-jaya*, conquest of the senses. This in turn brings speed of thought, independence in one's existence, and then *pradhāna-jaya*, conquest of the entire material sphere. It is here I think that we can see that Patañjali is turning his attention back to the subject of *kaivalya*, release from this world, which is achieved through *pradhāna-jaya*, mastery over matter.

This is confirmed in *sūtra* 49, which brings us to the point of *sattva-puruṣānyatā-khyāti*, the higher realisation of the nature of the self, which brings control over everything that exists, and knowledge of all things. One gets a clear sense here that the transition from discussing materialistic supernatural powers to a consideration of spiritual perfection is seamless and without any sense of conflict. The powers come, the *yogin* experiences them, and then he or she moves on to the higher level, which is the power to see beyond the world, and exist in terms of the true spiritual identity.

50–55: RENOUNCING THE POWERS AND ACHIEVING KAIVALYA

50. *tad-vairāgyād api doṣa-bīja-kṣaye kaivalyam,*
    And when, as a result of renouncing such powers, the seed of contamination dwindles, one attains *kaivalya*, separation from matter.

51. *sthāny-upanimantraṇe saṅga-smayākaraṇaṃ punar-aniṣṭa-prasaṅgāt,*
    If one receives invitations from higher beings, one should not take pleasure in such contacts, for they may again arouse unwanted attachments.

52. *kṣaṇa-tat-kramayoḥ saṁyamād viveka-jaṁ jñānam,*
Through *saṁyama* on instants of time and their sequence, one acquires the knowledge born of discrimination.

53. *jāti-lakṣaṇa-deśair anyatānavacchedāt tulyayos tataḥ pratipattiḥ,*
Then one gains the ability to properly perceive the two identical entities that cannot be distinguished by their birth, characteristics, or place.

54. *tārakaṃ sarva-viṣayaṁ sarvathā-viṣayam akramaṁ ceti viveka-jaṁ jñānam,*
The knowledge born of discrimination allows one to cross beyond the world, it includes all objects and all times, and is not confined to any form of sequential reasoning.

55. *sattva-puruṣayoḥ śuddhi-sāmye kaivalyam iti,*
When there is perfect balance between *sattva* and *puruṣa*, this is *kaivalya*.

It is in these final *sūtras* of the *Vibhūti-Pāda* that Patañjali wholly returns to his previous line of discussion, as he reveals how Yoga is to be used as a means to achieve spiritual rather than worldly goals. There is a quick transition here, as the text first notes that the powers indicated previously are to be renounced, *tad-vairāgyāt*, and attention shifted instead to the pursuit of *viveka-jaṁ jñānam*, the knowledge that arises when the power of discrimination is exercised. Knowledge of this type allows understanding of both *sattva* and *puruṣa*, and, crucially, discriminates between them, thereby dispelling the illusion that binds the soul. Only when *sattva* and *puruṣa* are returned to their true distinctive states can *kaivalya* be achieved, and the *puruṣa* attain liberation from rebirth.

Sūtra 50 begins with the phrase *tad-vairāgyāt*, by renouncing that, and here we must presume that the word *tat* (meaning that) refers to the absolute control over the world discussed in *sūtra* 49. In other words, it is only when the control of the world given through yogic *siddhis* is renounced that the higher goals of Yoga can be achieved. When this is done, the *doṣa-bīja*, the seed from which impurity sprouts, finally wastes away, and *kaivalya* becomes possible. Hence it is made clear that as long as there is any aspiration for the powers previously listed, a seed of impurity will remain as a barrier to *kaivalya*. *Sūtra* 51 then refers to the inducements offered by gods or higher beings, which, like the *siddhis*, must also be ignored. Here we are reminded of the numerous stories found in the *Purāṇas* and elsewhere in which Indra and the other Vedic gods try to break the vows of a great *yogin*, often by sending one of the voluptuous celestial women to allure and seduce the sage. The story of Viśvamitra, which first appears in the *Rāmāyaṇa*, comes particularly to mind.

By applying the art of *saṁyama* to the progression of time, one acquires a form of knowledge that arises out of *viveka*, the power of discrimination. The concept of *viveka* is a very important one in Indian religious thought, indicating as it does the ability to distinguish spirit from matter, and thereby transcend the false sense of identity that binds the soul to this world. Typically, we understand our identity in terms of the body and the mind, which are distinct from the *puruṣa*, but the knowledge born of discrimination allows us to see the truth of our identity. And when this knowledge is acquired, it becomes possible to understand both matter and spirit, *sattva* and *puruṣa*, as distinct from one another.

Sūtra 54 gives four characteristics of this *viveka-jaṁ jñānam*. It is *tāraka*, it is *sarva-viṣayam*, it is *sarvathā-viṣayam*, and it is *akramam*. *Tāraka* is often translated as intuitive or transcendent, and this is certainly possible, but I have chosen to read it in a more literal sense. *Tāraka* can sometimes mean a ferryman, and hence it may well indicate that knowledge of this type is the means by which we can be carried from a lower state of existence to *kaivalya*, the realm of the spirit. *Sarva-viṣaya* and *sarvathā-viṣaya* then indicate that this knowledge embraces all subjects in all places; in a similar way, Kṛṣṇa says in the *Bhagavad-gītā*, *yaj jñātvā neha bhūyo 'nyaj jñātavyam avaśiṣyate*, when this is known, nothing further remains to be known (7.2). And finally *akrama* indicates that this knowledge does not come step by step but is instantaneous, and I have taken this to mean that it is not derived from the mental thought process of sequential reasoning, but is a spontaneous realisation of the truth that arises as a natural consequence of profound *saṁyama.*

The final *sūtra* of the chapter then offers a definition of *kaivalya*, as *sattva-puruṣayoḥ śuddhi-sāmye*. Here again, *sattva* and *puruṣa* indicate matter and spirit, or the body and the soul, but śuddhi-*sāmye* is a little more difficult. It could mean 'when there is equal purity', but I am inclined to read it from a Sāṁkhya perspective, as indicating that both *sattva* and *puruṣa* exist in their pure states, or in other words without any mingling of the two principles. The usual meaning of *kaivalya* is 'being separate', or 'being alone', and hence it would be logical to take śuddhi-*sāmye* as indicating that each exists unaffected by the other.

These last *sūtras* of the *Vibhūti-Pāda* have laid the ground for the final section of Patañjali's teachings, which is entitled the *Kaivalya-Pāda*

CHAPTER 4: THE KAIVALYA-PĀDA

THE fourth and final chapter of the *Yoga Sūtras* is entitled the *Kaivalya-Pāda*, indicating that in this concluding section of his work Patañjali is turning to consider the ultimate goal of the practice and philosophy he has expounded up until this point. The word *kaivalya* is widely encountered in Indian religious literature, but it is particularly associated with Sāṁkhya discourse. It is derived from the word *kevala*, which means singly, exclusively, or alone, and *kaivalya* can hence be rendered as 'aloneness', or the state of being alone. What it really refers to is separation of *puruṣa* from *prakṭrti*, so that the soul no longer has to experience the misery and death that arise from this unwanted association. The Yoga system is offered by Patañjali as a means by which this separation of the soul from matter can be achieved, and the progression of rebirths brought to an end. In that sense it can be understood as a term broadly equivalent to *mokṣa* in Hindu thought, or *nirvāṇa* amongst Buddhists.

The chapter is not, however, the easiest to comprehend, and it requires careful consideration in order to understand exactly what Patañjali is saying here; and even then it is not always exactly clear. The opening section returns to a consideration of the doctrine of karma, exploring how and why it is that actions performed yield a future result, as one's personal destiny unfolds. The answer suggested here is that action is never lost as it creates a *saṁskāra*, or impression, on the consciousness; and it is this mental condition that actually produces the future result of action. Hence mental solutions can be applied to the problem of karma as the attempt is made to arrest the progression of action and reaction.

The middle *sūtras* of the chapter are probably the most difficult, as Patañjali attempts to explain the reality of the world we inhabit, and the way that perception, a mental process, shapes the nature of our personal reality. He is not quite saying that the world we live in is a mental creation, but he is saying that the reality we experience is profoundly influenced by the mode of perception. Hence mental adjustment, and a realignment of perception, can have a genuine effect on the reality in which we exist.

Then, from around *sūtra* 18 onwards, the focus of the discussion moves on to the nature of the *puruṣa*, the transcendent spiritual component of our being, referred to elsewhere as the *ātman*. The *puruṣa* exists as the very essence of what we are, but it cannot be perceived whilst the mind projects its perception outwards via the senses. And even if this outward projection can be suspended, there are still the *saṁskāras*, or latent impressions of previous experiences, that must be ended. The whole of Patañjali's Yoga system has been designed to accomplish this task of stilling the mind, suspending outward perception, and then gradually eroding the existing *saṁskāras*. Only if this can be achieved does the existence of *puruṣa* become apparent.

The final *sūtras* then indicate that it is this inward perception of the *puruṣa* that is the key to *kaivalya*, which occurs when material desires cease, when past *saṁskāras* are eroded, and when the state of *samādhi* is pure. At this point, the *puruṣa* attains its natural position, devoid of any contact with matter, and is no longer affected by the unwanted conditions of death and rebirth.

1–5: THE PROCESS OF REBIRTH

1. *janmauṣadhi-mantra-tapaḥ-samādhi-jāḥ siddhayaḥ,*
   The higher powers arise from birth, herbs, *mantras*, austerity, and achieving *samādhi*.

2. *jāty-antara-pariṇāmaḥ prakṛty-āpūrāt,*
The transformation into another birth is caused by the flooding over of that different nature.

3. *nimittam aprayojakaṁ prakṛtīnāṁ varaṇa-bhedas tu tataḥ kṣetrikavat,*
There is, however, no external cause that directly brings about these different natures. It is just like when a farmer breaks the field boundaries, allowing the water to take its natural course.

4. *nirmāṇa-cittāny asmitā-mātrāt,*
Differing mentalities are formed solely from the sense of 'I'-ness.

5. *pravṛtti-bhede prayojakaṁ cittam ekam anekeṣām,*
In the varying types of action performed by many different entities, it is the single element known as *citta*, mentality, that is the causal factor.

Here the opening verse is used to bring about a transition from one topic to the next. The *siddhis*, or mystical perfections, have been described in the previous chapter, and here it is said that in addition to *samādhi* such supernatural powers can also be gained through the use of herbs, *mantras*, acts of austerity, or simply due to one's birth. This idea of powers arising simply from birth is not entirely clear, but it probably means that some persons are born with such abilities.

This then provides a starting point for a discussion of birth and rebirth, and the factors that determine the nature of rebirth. Virtually all schools of Indian philosophy accept that the action a person performs will affect his or her future destiny, and will determine the nature of future births; this point has already been confirmed by Patañjali. Here, however, the process is considered in more detail, and some explanation is given as to how this law of karma operates. What the text seems to be asserting is firstly that there is no external force or deity overseeing the process, and secondly, that there is a close interaction between action, the fruit of action, and the mentality underlying the action.

On the first of these two points, it is sometimes thought that the law of karma is somewhat equivalent to the notion of divine justice encountered in Christianity or Islam. Here, however, this idea is rejected, as the progression from action performed to future consequences is compared to the flowing of water from a higher position to a lower one; in other words, it is a natural law of the universe, and is not dependent on the dispensation of some celestial judge and law maker. This occurs because every experience and every action leaves a latent impression upon the *citta*, so that an action does not end when its performance is complete. The mentality of the performer is transformed by the action, and it is this mental transformation wrought by action that causes the action to produce a future result, as the law of karma unfolds.

This point is significant for Yoga philosophy, because it means that the transformation of the *citta* that Yoga produces can have a direct effect on the nature of one's future existence in the world, and can in fact bring the chain of karmic reactions to an end.

6–8: THE EFFECTS OF YOGA ON KARMA

6. *tatra dhyāna-jam anāśayam,*
   But the mental state shaped by *dhyāna*, meditation, leaves no impression.

7. *karmāśuklākṛṣṇaṁ yoginas tri-vidham itareṣām,*
   Action performed by *yogins* is neither white nor black, but action performed by others is of three types.

8. *tatas tad-vipākānuguṇānām evābhivyaktir vāsanānām,*
   Latent impressions are formed as a result of these three types of action, and these ripen into the results that correspond to them.

Here the previous point is further elaborated upon, and related to the Yoga practice Patañjali has previously described. We have been told that the law of karma is based on the fact that actions leave a latent impression on the mind that later becomes manifest as the results of action. According to *sūtra* 6, however, the exception to this rule is *dhyāna*, meditation, which leaves no impression whatsoever. This point is clearly leading us in the direction of *kaivalya*, the main topic of the chapter, for if yogic action leaves no *saṁskāra* on the mind, then it will not produce any future reaction, and the progression of the law of karma will be interrupted.

Sūtra 7 reiterates the point. In line with the assertion of the *Bhagavad-gītā* (18.12), action is said to be of three types, which are described as being black, white and (one presumes) a mixture of the two. In other words, action can be righteous and produce a good result, wicked and produce an unwanted result, or else mixed and produce a mixed result. But the action of the *yogin* who absorbs himself in meditation transcends these categorisations and therefore transcends the law of karma. Actions that fall within the three categories produce latent impressions, and therefore we can quite reasonably infer that the action of the *yogin* that is outside these categories produces no *saṁskāras*, and hence in the language of the *Gītā* is *a-karma*.

Here I feel that we are very much in contact with the *Bhagavad-gītā*'s discourse on action and non-action (karma and *akarma*), which is to be found in its fourth chapter. There Kṛṣṇa reveals that it is not directly the action itself that produces the future result, but rather the state of consciousness that motivates the action. Hence if an action is performed without any desire or attachment, it is in fact *a-karma* because there is no future result. I think we can detect here that Patañjali is speaking along very similar lines in suggesting that yogic action transcends the law of karma because it is based on an alternative state of consciousness. It is in this way that the *yogin* can escape from the bondage of karma and achieve the ultimate goal of *kaivalya* and liberation from rebirth.

9–13: LATENT IMPRESSIONS AND THE RESULTS OF ACTION

9. *jāti-deśa-kāla-vyavahitānām apy ānantaryaṁ smṛti-saṁskārayor eka-rūpatvāt,*
   Although there may be separation in terms of birth, place, and time, because these impressions have a form identical to memory, they still remain in direct contact.

10. *tāsām anāditvaṁ cāśiṣo nityatvāt,*
    And because of the eternal nature of desire, these latent impressions have no beginning point.

11. *hetu-phalāśrayālambanaiḥ saṁgṛhītatvād eṣām abhāve tad-abhāvaḥ,*
    Because latent impressions are dependent upon the cause, the result, the foundation, and the support, if these cease to exist then the impressions will also be removed.

12. *atītānāgataṁ svarūpato 'sty adhva-bhedād dharmāṇām,*
    The reality of past and future is established because of the different directions in their essential nature.

13. *te vyakta-sūkṣmā-guṇātmānaḥ,*
    These are manifest and subtle, and are shaped by the *guṇas*.

Here Patañjali explains more about *saṁskāras*, the latent impressions left on the mind by action performed. *Sūtra* 9 explains again that an action performed has a permanent effect because of the *saṁskāra* it generates. These are compared to memories, for it is easy to see that an action persists within the mind in the form of our recollection of it, and in this sense the *saṁskāra* of an action can be regarded as a form of subtle memory. We might ask how the soul came to be in this position, and at what point it became afflicted by the burden of *saṁskāras* that lead in turn to karmic reactions and rebirth. As is often the case in Indian religious thought, the question is deflected by the assertion that it has no beginning because the desire that causes action, and hence *saṁskāras*, is without beginning.

In *sūtra* 11 it is stated that the *saṁskāras* have a cause and an effect as well as a foundation and a support, though precisely what these are is not explained. Patañjali's point here seems to be that the existence of *saṁskāras* can be tackled by removing the factors that shape them, the process of cause and effect, and the foundation upon which they rest. *Sūtra* 12 is rather obscure but seems to build upon the idea of *hetu* and *phala*, cause and result, noted in 11. The essential nature of past and future can be distinguished because of the different directions in which they move, which may be as simple as pointing out that the past is moving away from us whilst the future is moving towards us. And this of course ties in closely with the notion of karma, and the way an action creates a *saṁskāra* before retreating into the past, whilst the *saṁskāra* remains to create a result at some point in the future. Vyasa agrees with this interpretation, pointing out that the past is distinct from the future because in the past objects have attained a state of actual existence, whilst those in the future exist only in a potential state.

It is this point that is probably being referred to in *sūtra* 13 where the essential natures of past and future are described as being *vyakta*, manifest or visible, and *sūkṣma*, existing only in a subtle form. In both cases, however, they are *guṇātmaka*, composed of the *guṇas*, which are the essential qualities of matter. The idea that *prakṛti*, or matter, is imbued with three qualities, *sattva*, *rajas* and *tamas*, is one of the fundamental principles of Sāṁkhya doctrine, and is also a prominent feature of the teachings contained in the *Bhagavad-gītā* and the *Mahābhārata*. According to this notion, all facets of the material manifestation are shaped by a combination of these essential qualities. The terms themselves are very difficult to translate effectively, but broadly speaking *sattva* is truth, purity, light, goodness, and virtue, *rajas* is passion, energy, action, and achievement, and *tamas* is darkness, illusion, inertia, and impurity. Here Patañjali is asserting that despite the differences between the nature of past and future, all such manifestations fall within the domain of the *guṇas*, and hence stand outside the spiritual identity of the *puruṣa*.

14–17: OBJECTS AND THE PERCEPTION OF OBJECTS

14. *pariṇāmaikatvād vastu-tattvam,*
Because it retains a single identity through various transformations, there is reality to an object.

15. *vastu-sāmye citta-bhedāt tayor vibhaktaḥ panthāḥ,*
An object has the same identity in all circumstances, but due to differences of mentality between two persons, the paths of perception diverge.

16. *na caika-citta-tantraṁ vastu tad-apramāṇakaṁ tadā kiṁ syāt,*
An object cannot be shaped by one mind alone. If that were the case, what would happen if it were not perceived by that mind?

17. *tad-uparāgāpekṣitvāc cittasya vastu jñātājñātam,*
An object is either known or unknown by the mind

depending on the extent to which it colours the mind's perception.

In this passage, Patañjali explores some of the more subtle aspects of Indian philosophy, and in particular the reality or otherwise of this world. It is well known that Śaṅkarācārya made the statement, *brahma satyaṁ jagan mithyā*, Brahman is real but the world is an illusion, whilst the Buddhists held to śūnyavāda, a doctrine of emptiness, which taught that there is nothing permanent in the world and hence nothing that could be regarded as absolutely real. Śaṅkara's doctrine is different to that of the Buddhists in that he taught that there is absolute reality, which is Brahman, but the perception of that reality is distorted by the power of illusion (*māyā*), and is false. Hence his doctrine is sometimes referred to as a *māyāvāda*. Given the historical period in which Patañjali was writing, it seems likely that he is here rejecting the Buddhist śūnyavāda, since the *māyāvāda*, the doctrine of illusion, did not rise to prominence until several centuries later, following the writings of Gaudapāda and Śaṅkarācārya.

In this passage, the *Yoga Sūtras* confirms the Sāṁkhya *satyavāda*, which claims that the world we perceive is real. Our perception of it may be flawed, but each object does have an objective reality to it. *Sūtra* 14 proclaims the point very clearly. Despite the transformations of time, an object retains a single identity and hence *vastu-tattvam*, the object is real in the form perceived. The text then considers the significance of perception in relation to reality, for some might hold the view that the reality and nature of an object are contingent on the perception of it. Patañjali does not accept this idealist perspective. Different persons may have a different perception of an object, but the object itself retains an objective identity that transcends perception.

This point is then demonstrated in *sūtras* 16 and 17. If the nature of an object were contingent on perception, he asks rhetorically, what would be the nature of the object if it were outside the range of perception? Objects are sometimes perceived, and known, and sometimes they are not, but surely we cannot say that they cease to exist when they are not within the purview of mental perception? In this way, Patañjali rejects the notion of a purely subjective reality and insists that the world has an objective reality independent of perception.

18–23: THE MIND AND THE PURUṢA

18. *sadā jñātāś citta-vṛttayas tat-prabhoḥ puruṣasyāpariṇāmitvāt,*
The movements of the mind are always known to the *puruṣa*, the master of the mind. This is because the *puruṣa* is never subject to transformation.

19. *na tat svābhāsaṁ dṛśyatvāt,*
Because the mind is thus itself an object of perception, it cannot be regarded as self-illuminating.

20. *eka-samaye cobhayānavadhāraṇam,*
And it is unable to perceive both itself and its object at the same time.

21. *cittāntara-dṛśye buddhi-buddher atiprasaṅgaḥ smṛti-saṁkaraś ca,*
If one mind were subject to the perception of another, then one intellect would become inseparable from the other, and their memories would be mixed up.

22. *citer apratisaṁkramāyās tad-ākārāpattau sva-buddhi-saṁvedanam,*
But when the mind ceases its transformations, the *puruṣa* takes on its appearance, and then becomes conscious of its own intellect.

23. *draṣṭṛ-dṛśyoparaktaṃ cittaṃ sarvārtham,*
When the mind is thus coloured by both the seer and the seen, it becomes capable of perceiving all objects.

In this difficult and rather obscure passage, Patañjali appears now to be drawing a distinction between the *puruṣa*, the soul, the mind, and the world it perceives. Firstly, he insists that the *puruṣa* is never subject to transformation as the mind and the world are. Hence its inherent state of knowledge is unimpeded, and it is able to know both the *citta* and its *vṛtti*, its wandering thought processes. Here it seems that Patañjali is trying to show that the knowledge inherent within the *puruṣa* is different from the knowledge acquired through mental processes, which is incomplete and prone to misapprehension. Moreover, the mind is dependent upon *puruṣa*, and is itself known to the *puruṣa*; hence it is not to be regarded as an independent knower, but rather as a tool or reflection of the *puruṣa*.

Whilst the mind is perceiving an external object, it cannot be aware of its own identity, and hence the domain of its knowledge is inhibited and partial, the implication being that the knowledge inherent within the *puruṣa* is absolute. If it were possible for the mind to be aware of thought processes, then distinctive memories would become confused and mixed together; this assertion in *sūtra* 21 is not entirely clear, but Vyasa regards it as a further argument through which Patañjali is seeking to refute the Buddhist position on reality and perception.

The real crux of the passage would seem to come in 22 where we are abruptly brought back to Yoga discourse. It is only when the transformations of the mind are suspended that these limitations on the thought processes can be overcome. How is this? At this point the *puruṣa* itself assumes the identity of the mind bringing with it its own unique powers of perception. This is clearly the result sought through Yoga practice, arising as it does from *citta-vṛtti-nirodha,* the suspension of the movements of the mind. When this is achieved, the mental processes are no longer solely directed outwards through sensory perception of the world (here referred to as *dṛśya*, that which is perceived), for a consciousness of the *draṣṭṛ*, the seer, also arises.

Now we start to see where Patañjali is going with this discussion, as he begins to draw it back towards the point from which he began. The wanderings of the mind, as it perceives the world through the senses, are to be restrained, for only then does the existence of the *puruṣa* begin to become manifest. The cause of bondage, illusion, and rebirth, is *avidyā*, a lack of true knowledge, but the Yoga system is here shown to be addressing that condition in such a way that full knowledge, including knowledge of the *puruṣa*, arises within the practitioner. This then is the gateway to *kaivalya*, separation from matter, and the cessation of continual rebirth, and this is the conclusion towards which Patañjali is now seeking to draw his readers.

24–28: APPROACHING KAIVALYA

24. *tad-asaṁkhyeya-vāsanābhiś citram api parārthaṃ saṁhatya-kāritvāt,*
Although the mind becomes variegated due to the influence of the countless impressions it bears, it is now acting in combination with the other, and thus serves the other's purpose.

25. *viśeṣa-darśina ātma-bhāva-bhāvanā-vinivṛttiḥ,*
A person who can perceive the distinction puts an end to the condition that causes his own existence.

26. *tadā viveka-nimnaṁ kaivalya-prāg-bhāraṁ cittam,*
Then, by immersion in discriminative understanding, the main bulk of the mind moves towards *kaivalya.*

27. *tac-chidreṣu pratyayāntarāṇi saṁskārebhyaḥ,*
When this state is disrupted, other conceptualisations emerge as a result of existing latent impressions.

28. *hānam eṣāṁ kleśavad uktam,*
It is said that these can be negated in the same manner as the afflictions mentioned earlier.

At this point the final conclusion to the *Yoga Sūtras* is clearly in sight. The previous passage arrived at the point where the thought processes, the *citta*, are no longer directed solely outwards, but are able to operate in relation to the *draṣṭṛ*, the soul that perceives, as well as the *dṛśya*, the world that is perceived. However, the *saṁskāras* or *vāsanās*, the latent impressions left on the consciousness by previous actions, are still present and can obstruct the higher realisation that the Yoga practice is beginning to yield. But the mind is now acting on behalf of the other, the *puruṣa*, and is combined with the *puruṣa*, so that even the latent impressions cannot have their previous effect.

Thus the *yogin* becomes *viśeṣa-darśin,* able to perceive the distinction between the *puruṣa* and the world, and through this perception he is able to bring about the cessation of repeated existence. So here again, in *sūtra* 25, Patañjali is revealing that the true purpose of the Yoga system he is teaching is to put an end to existence in this world, and to the chain of karmic reactions that perpetuates this existence. At this point, the *yogin* is absorbed in *viveka*, the discriminative insight that grants knowledge of her true self, and as a result the *citta* moves away from this world and towards *kaivalya*, the state of separation from it.

This process is not yet complete, however, and the *saṁskāras* can still prove to be an obstruction in the progression of the consciousness towards *kaivalya*. When this occurs, Patañajali advises that the *saṁskāras* be dealt with in the same way as was recommended earlier with regard to the *kleśas*, the obstacles or afflictions. Here the text is clearly referring back to *sūtra* 32 of the first chapter where *eka tattva abhyāsa*, regular practice in relation to a single object, was recommended as the means by which the *kleśas* can be nullified. Here therefore the same method is being recommended for dealing with the remaining *saṁskāras*, which may still inhibit the adept's progress towards *kaivalya.*

29–34: ACHIEVING KAIVALYA

29. *prasaṁkhyāne 'py akusīdasya sarvathā viveka-khyāter dharma-meghaḥ samādhiḥ,*
For one who seeks nothing at all, even though he has reached an elevated position through his discriminative insight, the *dharma* cloud of *samādhi* then appears.

30. *tataḥ kleśa-karma-nivṛttiḥ,*
And as a result the afflictions and the influence of karma cease to be active.

31. *tadā sarvāvaraṇa-malāpetasya jñānasyānantyāj jñeyam alpam,*
For such a person, who has had the entire covering of impurity removed, there then remains little further to be known, because of the unlimited nature of the knowledge he has realised.

32. *tataḥ kṛtārthānāṁ pariṇāma-krama-samāptir guṇānām,*
Then the sequential movement of the *guṇas* from one to the other comes to an end, for they have fulfilled their purpose.

33. *kṣaṇa-pratiyogī pariṇāmāparānta-nirgrāhyaḥ kramaḥ,*

The sequence of movement takes place moment by moment, but is perceived only at the end of the transformations.

34. *puruṣārtha-śūnyānāṁ guṇānāṁ pratiprasavaḥ kaivalyaṁ svarūpa-praviṣṭhā vā citi-śaktir iti,* *Kaivalya* means to inhibit the flow of the *guṇas,* which have no purpose for the *puruṣa.* Or it can be said to be the potency of the true consciousness when it achieves its natural condition.

In these final *sūtras,* Patañjali brings his discourse to a conclusion by revealing the ultimate goal that can be achieved through Yoga practice, which he names again as *kaivalya.* Here then it is explained what is meant by *kaivalya,* and how this most elevated state of existence is finally achieved.

Firstly, it is available only to one who renounces all desire for success in this world, and we must presume that this refers to the magical powers described in Chapter 3. Then for one who has achieved *viveka-khyāti,* discriminative knowledge, the dharma cloud of *samādhi* becomes manifest. *Viveka-khyāti* must here refer to the power to discriminate between soul and matter, so that one no longer sees oneself in terms of the present identity; rather one understands that the transcendent *puruṣa,* untouched by matter, is the true self. The phrase *dharma-megha-samādhi* may be a metaphor invoking the clouds that appear during the monsoon season; such clouds are filled with rain, but here they are described as dharma clouds. Today the word dharma is usually understood as virtue, duty, or proper conduct, and Vyasa takes it in that sense in his commentary on this *sūtra,* suggesting that the realised *yogin* is inherently virtuous because he no longer sees the world in terms of the body and mind. Dharma, however, also has the meaning of 'inherent nature', and it may be that Patañjali is suggesting that the state of *samādhi* brings full consciousness of one's true spiritual identity, rather than identifying oneself in terms of body and mind.

When this *dharma-megha-samādhi* appears to the adept, karma and *kleśa* both cease. This short *sūtra* 30 has a very profound message, for it has already been explained how karma perpetuates our existence in this world. When the appearance of *dharma-megha-samādhi* ends the chain of reactions, then rebirth and material existence must also cease. The word *kleśa* might refer to the obstacles to Yoga practice previously considered, but it might also be used in a more general sense to indicate that the miseries of life, such as old age, disease, and death, also come to an end alongside the cessation of karmic reactions.

It is then further revealed that in this state of realisation, *jñeyam alpam*, there is very little that is left to be known, a statement that is notably similar to one found in the *Bhagavad-gītā*, where Kṛṣṇa asserts, *yaj jñātvā* neha bhūyo 'nyaj jñātavyam avaśiṣ*yate*, 'when this is known, nothing else remains to be known' (7.2). The state of *samādhi* brings absolute knowledge of the world so that one can clearly recognise the nature of matter and the way in which *puruṣa* is distinct from matter. In our normal condition, knowledge is limited because we perceive through the senses, and are only aware of the external world. The experience of *samādhi*, however, allows these conventional limits of knowledge to be transcended, so that the *jñāna* is *ānantya*, without limitation.

Sūtra 32 refers again to the action of the three *guṇas*. When *kaivalya* is attained, the movement of the *guṇas* ceases, and they are said to have fulfilled their function. Here one needs to refer to the Sāṁkhya teaching about the way in which *prakṛti*, matter, begins to evolve from a non-manifest state into the variegated forms the world is composed of. This process of evolution is set in motion by the *guṇas* becoming active, and not remaining in a state of balance. Here it is suggested that *samādhi* returns the *guṇas* to their prior state of balance, and thereby causes the action of *prakṛti* to cease.

The phrase *kṛtārtham*, with their function fulfilled, again confirms the view that the evolved state of matter appears solely to allow the *puruṣa* to gain its natural state of *kaivalya*. When this is achieved, the function of the *guṇas* is fulfilled, at least for that individual, and hence their movement is no longer required. The movement of the *guṇas* is a perpetual process for the living beings of this world, but it is only when the knowledge granted by *samādhi* is attained that one becomes aware of the true nature of one's own existence, for at this point, *jñeyam alpam*, there is very little that is still to be known.

In the final *sūtra*, Patañjali concludes his great work with a dual definition of *kaivalya*, the goal towards which his Yoga system is working. Firstly it is the state described in the previous *sūtra* in which the flow of the *guṇas* is finally suspended. In other words, it means the cessation of the *puruṣa*'s ignorance, and entanglement in matter. *Puruṣa* in its pure state has no need of *prakṛti*, or the *guṇas* of which *prakṛti* is comprised, and so when *kaivalya* is achieved the connection with the *guṇas* is discarded. This is one definition. Secondly, *kaivalya* can also be understood as the state of being in which the power of consciousness, the *citi-śakti*, returns to its original, natural state. This is a slightly more difficult concept, but it seems to indicate that the illusion of identifying with the body is discarded and replaced by the true understanding of one's identity as *puruṣa*. *Kaivalya* can thus also be understood as the attainment of knowledge of one's true spiritual identity. Thus Patañjali concludes his *Yoga Sūtras* by revealing again the real purpose behind his teachings, and thereby placing them within the mainstream of Indian religious and philosophical thought. As in Buddhism, Jainism, Vedānta, and Sāṁkhya, existence in this world, and the process of rebirth, is seen in a negative light, and the prospect of liberation from rebirth is held up as the highest goal. And as with these other systems, Patañjali is primarily concerned to explain the position of the true self, and to offer a practical technique through which this release can be attained.

CONCLUSIONS

THIS study of the *Yoga Sūtras* should have highlighted the main points of Patañjali's teaching, but it might be a good idea to conclude by drawing attention to a few of the principal ideas we have encountered, and perhaps considering what they reveal about the nature of Yoga as a whole. I will try to do this as briefly as possible so as to avoid too much repetition of points that have already been covered.

In terms of the context of the *Yoga Sūtras*, it seems apparent that the ideas encountered here are closely approximate to those found in the *Mahābhārata*, and especially in the *Bhagavad-gītā*. It cannot of course be proven in any way, but my strong instinct is that Patañjali was very much aware of the *Gītā*'s teachings, and in a number of places makes effective use of its ideas in structuring his own discourse. We have earlier alluded to the notion of a 'classical Yoga' distinct from the later Tantric practices, and if such a phenomenon does exist then we would probably include under that heading passages from the *Upaniṣads, Gītā,* and *Mahābhārata*, as well as the *Yoga Sūtras* itself.

Some, of course, will question the notion of a division between classical and later Yoga by arguing that Patañjali's awareness of *āsana* and *prāṇāyāma* shows that his ideas include the later forms, even if he does not elaborate on such practices in detail. It is certainly the case that the terse style of the *Yoga Sūtras* means that it does not go into any form of elaborate discussion, but nonetheless it is hard to deny that there is a fairly clear distinction between the Yoga philosophy advocated by Patañjali and the forms of Yoga widely practised today, particularly in the Western world.

If we were to try to define exactly what the *Yoga Sūtras* is saying we would have to conclude that its main concern is with a Yoga of the mind, and that the manipulation of the body is a relatively minor concern. Moreover, it is clearly apparent that this is a spiritual science that is closely aligned with Indian religious thought; indeed it is virtually impossible to separate the *Yoga Sūtras* from that context. Hence what we have here is a technique designed to bring the mental faculty under the volitional control of the practitioner so that the spiritual goal of liberation from rebirth can be attained. This, no more and no less, is what Patañjali is aiming to offer his students.

Hence the question may legitimately be raised as to the extent to which Patañjali should be regarded as the founder of the contemporary Yoga systems in which bodily manipulation receives so much emphasis. There is little doubt that many facets of contemporary practice are not derived from Patañjali, and therefore we do need to be cautious about proclaiming him to be the father of Yoga. On the other hand, it would be equally wrong to dismiss his role entirely. Perhaps it would be best to say that Patañjali devised a core system of Yoga practice that has been built upon, extended, and reinterpreted over the succeeding centuries so that the Yoga we are familiar with today is very different from that of Patañjali's vision, but at the same time not entirely distinct from it.

So where have these modifications and developments come from? A study of Indian religion reveals that soon after about 400 AD, the traditional Vedic, Buddhist, and Jain traditions became increasingly influenced by Tantric ideas, which may have equally ancient antecedents, but which probably existed outside the domain of Sanskrit culture prior to this period. Over the succeeding centuries these more orthodox traditions began to absorb more and more elements of Tantric belief and practice until this became their principal rather than their marginal identity. Hence I think we can safely conclude that this same process of Tantricisation applied to the Yoga tradition just as much as it did to other areas of Indian spirituality, so that the original forms of Yoga practice we encounter in the *Yoga Sūtras*, *Bhagavad-gītā* and elsewhere became increasingly overlaid with the Tantric practices that predominate in contemporary Yoga.

Lightning Source UK Ltd.
Milton Keynes UK
UKHW021833220119
336023UK00029B/1486/P

9 781527 210370